How To Have Twins
Double The Fun!

How I PLANNED to have my identical twin girls naturally.

Includes how to increase your chances of getting pregnant/having twins/having girls/having boys.

by

Gale Glenbury

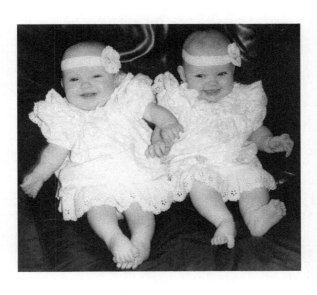

Table of Contents

Table of Contents

Foreword

So, I guess you would like to have twins, as you've bought this book! Great! You and your partner want to be the proud parents of twins!

I have wanted to write this book for 21 years, when my twin girls were born. I am so glad I did.

Why am I writing it now, I hear you ask? Well, my identical twin girls are now 21 and they have always told me they want twins too. As twins do not run in my family, I advised them to practice what I did, as it worked for me, so perhaps it might work for them. Rather than saying it, I decided to put it all in writing. Maybe in a few years time, I will be a grandma of 2 pairs of twins. How wonderful would that be!

This book is written with 3 goals in mind:

1) To help my twins to have twins, if they still want twins when they are ready for children.

2) To help people, like yourself, to have twins.

3) An "ode" to my twin daughters to tell them how much they mean to us parents.

Each time I tell my story to people and how I planned to have twins, they are totally shocked and amazed.

I hope I will help all women who would like to have twins to make it a reality. Since I was 16, I dreamt of having identical twin girls. I just knew I was going to have them! 21 years ago, that dream came true.

Important, please read:

Almost none of the methods in this book are scientifically proven and are based on research. Please be aware that there is absolutely no guarantee that you will either get pregnant or have twins even if you practice every single method in this book.

It worked for me; you will read which methods I practiced towards the end of this book. If it worked for me, I see no reason at all why it wouldn't work for you. Some of these methods might work for some; others might not work at all.

This book is the end result of my research. Yes, you can find all the information in this book yourself in all different places, but if you are like me, you want everything you need to know to be in one place, bundled together, for your convenience. That's probably why you are reading this book.

When I did my research, 22 years ago, when I wanted to get pregnant, there was little available online as the Internet was not as big as it is now. I used to read books and talk to professionals.

All the photographs in this book and on the cover, are my twin daughters, just in case you wondered. I have written a little bit of information *in Italics underneath each picture.*

I hope you will enjoy reading this book and more importantly, I hope some methods might work for you.

If you will indeed conceive twins, as a result of reading this book, that would be fantastic! I would be really happy to hear from you, so please contact me to tell me your story!

You can contact me by email to tell me your story or for any other remarks about this book.

You can email me at <u>howtohavetwins@gmail.com</u>

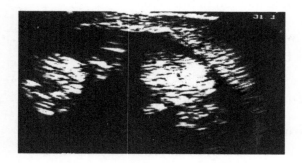

My first ultrasound: my babies at only a few weeks old.

Acknowledgements

Thank you to my husband for believing in me when I told him I wanted twins and I thought I knew how we were going to have them.

Lots of husbands would have laughed at the idea but you, my dear husband, believed in me. Even better - you did everything I asked you to do to maximise our chances. Without you, of course, we would not have had twins. We have had 21 very happy years with our two daughters and we have many more years to come! You are my life. I love you more than words can say.

Thank you Amelia and Sandra, my two identical twin daughters. You are my dream come true. You are beautiful, loving, happy, funny, helpful and intelligent young women.

(My daughters were bilingual at the age of 6 as I educated them with two languages. My husband would only speak English to them and I would only speak Flemish (my mother tongue) to them. Flemish by the way is like Dutch when written but pronounced differently. It is spoken in Belgium, where I am from).

We will never forget the endless hours of fun we had of the sound of you two giggling, joking, laughing and speaking your own language to each other. Not to mention the brilliant shows you used to perform for us!

Thank you for being such respectful young adults. I love you with all my heart. Everything I do, I do for you.

Chapter 1) The ever fascinating twins

1) Twins make the world go round

Twins are two babies, born usually within minutes of each other, and born from the same womb. How fascinating! Twins have been a talked about phenomenon for centuries and even today, many people believe there is something very physically special about them. Do they think the same thoughts? Do they eat the same foods? How are they connected?

Whenever most people see a set of twins, they can't help but stare. It is beyond fascinating and it is a common curiosity. I have always wanted to have twins and to experience all of the magical things that seem to go hand-in-hand with simply being around them.

This book is intended to give you the ins and outs of increasing your chances of having twins and at the same time, give you an inside view of the trials, and mostly, tribulations of having them.

I am still so pleased that I followed my instincts and research to create my personal formula for success. I am thrilled to be able to share it. Although, please keep in mind that many of these methods are not tried and tested. I feel that my success was due to using a combination of several methods that I personally believed in.

I hope you'll keep an open mind and try the methods and suggestions that resonate with you and your lifestyle.
Before we get started with all of the twin details, I thought you might enjoy a few twin statistics and facts to get you in the mood for all of the following information.

2) Interesting twin statistics

- Only 1 in 250 pregnancies result in **identical** twins.
- 4.5 million twins live in the United States.
- You are 3-4 times likely to have twins again if you have already had fraternal twins.
- Hispanics (Spanish) are less likely to birth twins
- China, with its enormous population, has one of the lowest birth rates of twins.
- Approximately 20 percent of twin births are to mothers over the age of 45.
- Conversely, only about 2 percent of teen pregnancies result in twins.
- Even with today's technology, almost 25 percent of twin births are unexpected.
- The average birth weight of twins is 5 lbs, 5 oz.
- The number of twin births in the U.S. has risen by 76 percent between 1980 and 2009, according to the National Centre for Health Statistics. The number of triplets has also increased.
- Generally, only the more developed countries have kept good birth records in the past, so less concrete information is available for some Asian countries.
- Although based on compiled information from this same study, it cites the African region as having some of the highest incidences of twin births. **Hispanic and Asian people have the lowest chance of having twins.**

3) Amusing and amazing twin facts

Some of these may seem a little far-fetched, but from my experience and also from research that has been done, the twin connection is strong. Being the mother of a set has confirmed my suspicions, and made me a believer.

- Twins account for over 90 percent of all multiple births.
- According to a study by the University of Padova, Italy, twins start playing and interacting at 14 weeks.
- George Mason and Bryan Caplan deduced from their study that separated twins still end up similar, possibly due to genetics.
- Twins can have separate dads! It has happened in 1-2 percent of twin births, where separate embryos were fertilized by two different men! Obviously, intercourse with both men would have happened within a relatively short period of time.
- Identical twins have the same DNA, but don't have the same fingerprints.
- More than double the amount of single births, twins have a 22 percent chance of being left-handed.
- Twin-speak is not a fallacy. Research by the General Linguistics journal states that twins are able to communicate by using their own language.
- It is an old wives tale that twin births skip a generation.
- Approximately one in three twins that are born are identical.
- About 25 percent of identical twins are mirror images of one another.
- Mothers of twins live longer, according to a University of Utah study that reviewed 59,000 cases between 1800 and 1970. That's always a good thing, right?

Some terminology:

Monozygotic – multiple (typically two) foetuses produced by the splitting of a single zygote.

Dizygotic – multiple (typically two) foetuses produced by two zygotes.

Polyzygotic – multiple foetuses produced by two or more zygotes.

Terms used for the order of multiple birth:

- Two offspring – twins
- Three offspring – triplets
- Four offspring – quadruplets
- Five offspring – quintuplets
- Six offspring – sextuplets
- Seven offspring – septuplets
- Eight offspring – octuplets
- Nine offspring – nonuplets
- Ten offspring – decaplets
- Eleven offspring – undecaplets
- Twelve offspring – duodecaplets

Chapter 2) What is a twin pregnancy?

1) Twins are a biological miracle

Having twin girls is something I always dreamed of, yet I knew, based on my family's history and all I'd been told, that it wasn't likely to happen.

Since it has been a high priority in my life, I started gathering information well before I was ready to conceive and as you know, my dreams became a reality! I knew fertility drugs were not for me, although I do include information on this in case it is something you wish to consider.

We all learnt the details of how twins are conceived in school, but until now never really needed to recall that information. As you know, there are different types of twins, fraternal and identical. It's the process that determines which type you may have. The biggest difference is that identical twins are always the same sex, while fraternal twins can be the same or one of each sex.
A pregnancy that has two or more foetuses is called a multiple pregnancy. Multiple foetuses can be the same or different; so identical or fraternal.

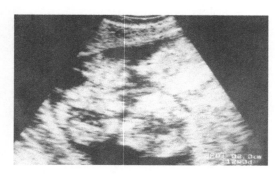

My ultrasound scan when my girls were only 12 weeks old.

2) Twins: Biology 101

Although you may not really have a preference about which type of twins you want, it's helpful to know the differences in how they are conceived. I'm convinced there are tricks that can help skew the results one way or the other, which we will discuss later.

3) We all know how to make a baby, right?

We all know that a baby comes from an intimate sexual encounter between a man and woman. It seems as though it is a simple matter of the male ejaculating his sperm into the vagina. Then the determined group of sperm rigorously swims into the vaginal canal in an attempt to reach and penetrate the egg that was recently released from the ovary.

Well, creating twins is the same process, except for one of the two following things takes place.

4) Identical twins

In biology class, we were taught that these identical beings were called monozygotic, which means they come from a split zygote, which forms two tiny embryos from one egg and one sperm. What that means is that one sperm fertilized one egg, and that egg split into two identical eggs, which produces two "identical" babies, the same gender.

Why this happens is not completely known. When this happens is somewhat interesting. It is during the first 4-14 days where the zygote actually splits into two smaller cells and they start growing independent of one another. Identical twins are random and not hereditary.

The scientific details are amazing and possibly too complicated to keep your interest. So let's move on to the whole fraternal twin phenomenon, which happens by a completely different process.

Some identical twins share the same placenta but mostly a separate amniotic sac grows in the womb. Very rarely do identical twins share one amniotic sac. Fraternal twins have separate placentas and separate amniotic sacs.

- Identical twins are always the same blood type and sex.

- Identical twins are NOT related to your age, family history or race.

- One might be right-handed and the other left-handed.

- One might look slightly different to the other, although they are called identical twins.

5) Fraternal twins

You can probably guess that fraternal twins are dizygotic, which means that two embryos develop from two eggs and two sperm. What happens here is that two lucky sperm find their way into two unsuspecting eggs. Fraternal twins are non-identical twins. Fraternal twins are the most common type of twins, where the mum has two eggs that are independently fertilised in the womb. The fertilisation is done by two different sperm cells from the father. Fraternal twins are genetically the same as any other babies. So in a way, you could say that fraternal twins are just siblings that are the same age.

This is so different from the identical twin process - yet, just as unique. The odds of two eggs being available for fertilization are as high as two sperm successfully penetrating the two eggs.

The children that are produced are twins, for sure, but not in the same way. They are almost more like siblings born at the same time, as they never shared the same cell, or DNA.

Both processes are always being studied because even after all of this time, there are some unknown mysteries.

- Fraternal twins can have different blood types and can be different sexes

- Fraternal twins ARE related to family history.

- Fraternal twins can look totally different from each other e.g. hair colour, eyes, ears, etc. but they can also look alike.

6) Semi Identical Twins

When two sperm cells fuse with a single egg, before becoming two embryos, semi-identical twins are formed. If the embryo survives, the result would be a set of twins with identical genes from the mother but different genes from the father's side. Semi-identical twins usually don't survive. However, a few rare cases are known to have survived.

7) Conceiving children relies on several factors

Remember, the time of the month, sperm count and other factors must be present for the sperm to be successful enough to fertilize the egg and create an embryo.

It's important to talk about all of these factors.

Chapter 3) Your body and pregnancy

A word about X and Y chromosomes

Chromosomes are tiny threadlike structures that each carry about 2,000 genes. Genes determine a baby's inherited characteristics, such as hair and eye colour, blood group, height and build.

A fertilised egg contains one sex chromosome from its mother and one from its father. The sex chromosome from the mother's egg is always the same and is known as the X chromosome. But the sex chromosome from the father's sperm may be an X or a Y chromosome.

If the egg is fertilised by a sperm containing an X chromosome, the baby will be a girl (XX). If the sperm contains a Y chromosome, the baby will be a boy (XY).

A word about ovulation

For most women, there are only 7 very fertile days in a month when you maximise your chances of getting pregnant: 6 days before you ovulate and the day of ovulation. 24 hours after ovulation you are too late and you've missed your most fertile time of the month.

Probability of Pregnancy from Intercourse on Days Relative to Ovulation

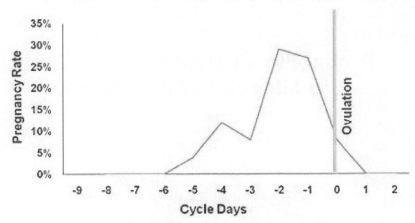

Source: www.cyclebeads.com

Some say you can get pregnant any day of your cycle, so be warned.

Every month, because of the hormonal changes in a woman's body, an egg is released from the ovaries. That egg travels through the fallopian tube into the womb. This is called ovulation. A woman cannot ovulate more than once during a cycle. Sperm can survive in the body for up to seven days after you've had sex. The menstrual cycle happens in 3 phases:
- Your body prepares to ovulate
- Ovulation happens
- Menstruation begins if that month's egg hasn't been fertilised. Having sex at the same time as the egg is released gives you the very best chances of getting pregnant.

To find out when you ovulate, subtract 14 days from the length of your monthly cycle, your cycle being the amount of days between your periods. Ovulation happens about 14 days before the first day of your period.

If you have a 28-day cycle, you will ovulate around day 14.

If you have a 25-day cycle, you will ovulate around day 11.

If you have a 35-day cycle, you will ovulate around day 21.

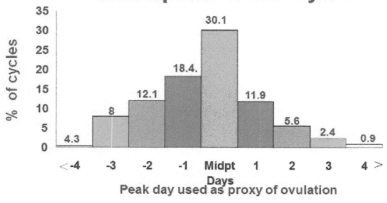

Probability of Ovulation Relative to Midpoint of the Cycle

Peak day used as proxy of ovulation

Source: IRH analysis of WHO 1981 data

After a woman ovulates, the egg will survive for only approx. 24 hours, but sperm can live up to 5/6 days. This is how you can increase your chances of getting pregnant two to three days before you ovulate. Don't wait to have sex until the day you ovulate as a man's sperm lives longer than a woman's egg. This means that an egg is often fertilised by sperm that has been in your body a few days before your egg was released. For you to get pregnant, a sperm must fertilise your egg.

Cyclebeads.com says: The Standard Day Method identifies 8 to 19 days as the potentially fertile days for women with cycles between 26 and 32 days long. This fertile window takes into account the variation in the timing of ovulation from one cycle to the next, the life span of the sperm and ovum, as well as the cycle length for the majority of women.

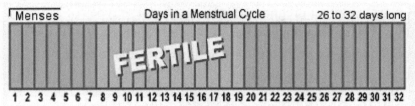

Signs of ovulation
Some women notice one of these signs, other women notice them all. Here are the signs of ovulation:
- Change in cervical fluid
- Light spotting
- Increase in your sex drive
- Abdominal bloating
- Dull ache or brief pain, felt on one side of your abdomen
- Body temperature that shows a clear change
- Tender breasts
- Heightened sense of smell or taste

1) How fertile is your body?

According to the latest buzz on pregnancy studies, there are definitely ways to increase fertility for both men and women. Some seem more complicated than others and none are tried and tested.

Before trying any of the methods that I've compiled from hundreds of sources, it is important that you and your partner take the time to visit a physician to make sure that you are both excellent pregnancy candidates to begin with.

There are tests and kits on the market to find out what your most fertile days of the month are called ovulation predictor kits. When I was trying to get pregnant, 22 years ago, these types of kits didn't exist or were known not to be very reliable.

So, instead of finding your most fertile days "the manual way", you can buy one of these kits.

2) A trip to your doctor will get you started

After all these years, you have a good idea of your own regularity and what is natural for your body.

You might be someone who has consistently regular periods that show up every 23 days. Alternatively, you could be a woman whose period varies each month. The length of the period generally lasts between three to five days, but there are those few who have daylong periods and others who have periods that seem to go on forever.

The first half of your cycle is when your oestrogen levels begin to rise. It's what makes the lining of the womb thicken, an environment that is ideal for nourishing a tiny embryo, should a pregnancy transpire.

If the egg is fertilized, it will attach itself to the uterine wall and begin the gestation process.

It is this process that we want to encourage.

If you have had a history of irregular periods, abnormal bleeding, severe pain, lack of periods or anything that seems suspicious, you definitely want to talk to your doctor and see if any of these symptoms are having any effect on your ability to conceive.

3) Fertility

You might be surprised that I am bringing this up, but don't be. Did you know that in about 40 percent of infertile couples, the man is a contributing factor? In fact, low sperm count makes up for about one-third of a couples' inability to get pregnant.

I hope that your man is on-board and willing to go the distance to make this pregnancy happen. I was lucky!

a) Check up and sperm tests

He will want to make an appointment with his urologist for a check-up and sperm tests. The sperm tests will review his sperm count, shape, movement and to see if there are any abnormalities worth noting. A hormone evaluation is also standard for checking testosterone, which is the leader of sperm production.

b) Basic questions about sexual lifestyle

He will be asked questions about exercise, sexual performance issues and if he has a history of any sexually transmitted diseases.

c) Genetic testing

Lastly, he may also undergo some genetic testing, which will look into his DNA to see if there are any mutations or information that will help determine the cause or probability of infertility.

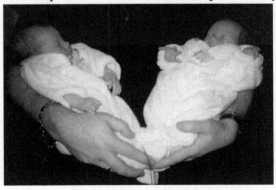

Me holding my precious little babies, a few months old.

Chapter 4) A few risks to be aware of

If you speak to parents of twins, they will have so much feedback your head will spin. Although we have all experienced many of the same things, there are always a few unique experiences that you'll figure out for yourself.

I'm sure that you realize that having two babies at the same time comes with extra work. Actually, you can expect extra everything with twins, just like you would with two children - except all at the same time.

Although I'm covering health risks, please realize that I am not trying to scare you, just making sure you are informed. Remember, risks imply there is the potential for danger, nothing more. All aspects of life have risks so keep that in mind. Walking across a busy street has risks. Weighing risk to reward is the bottom line. For me, the reward was so great that the risks were not on my mind during the entire pregnancy, although I took precautions.

So before I talk about how to increase your chances of having twins, I will talk about the negative sides first, just so you are aware of it all.

All multiple pregnancies increase complications and potential health risks. **To be aware is to be prepared.** Once you know what could happen, you will do your best to avoid some of the preventable issues.

a) Preeclampsia and eclampsia

Preeclampsia is a high blood pressure condition and a high level of protein in the urine. This condition can be serious and usually occurs during the second half of the pregnancy term.

The medical community isn't sure what causes this, but they suspect it may be problems with nutrition, high BMI (Body Mass Index), genetics and poor blood circulation. I will explain BMI later.

Watch out for these symptoms:
- swollen feet, legs and hands
- abdominal pain
- change in reflex response rate
- vomiting and/or nausea
- severe headaches
- dizziness
- blurry eyesight and sudden eye floaters

If untreated, it can turn into eclampsia, which is serious enough to increase the chances of death. With two babies at risk, you want to make sure to avoid this condition.

It often occurs in first-time pregnancies. To reduce the incidence, have your blood pressure checked regularly.

My twin girls were born 4 weeks premature because of eclampsia. My doctor told me it was best for the babies and for me to have a caesarean.

b) Protein-urea

Urinary protein excretion increases quite a bit during uncomplicated single pregnancies. It makes sense that the chances are increased with two pregnancies. Too much protein in the urine means potential damage to the kidneys and also the possibility of ending up with diabetes.

There are no symptoms that can be spotted in advance, other than swollen hands, feet and legs. Regular urine testing will help to find this condition.

c) Renal insufficiency and failure

Although this is a rare complication, the incidence is higher for twin pregnancies. Kidney failure or renal blockage can result in serious levels of waste and fluid that back up in the system. If this goes undetected or untreated, it could end up in chronic kidney disease - which could result in having to have dialysis or a kidney transplant.

d) Liver disease

Acute fatty liver is more common with twin pregnancies and is said to come up during the 35th or 36th week of pregnancy. It can be life threatening and so is worth mentioning. The cause might be the improper metabolism of fatty acids. With early detection, it can be reversed.

e) Antepartum hemorrhage

This is a fancy name for vaginal bleeding during the pregnancy. If it is going to happen, it is usually around the 20-24 weeks mark. Whether painful or not, this is not a normal condition and should be considered an emergency. It could lead to death for you and/or your twins. Don't take this lightly.

f) Abnormal umbilical artery

This is a fairly common occurrence and happens to 1 in 500 pregnant women. It is found more frequently in multiple births. Most umbilical cords have one vein and two arteries. In some cases, there is only one artery, which can be dangerous. In 75 percent of the cases, the babies are healthy and fine. In the remaining 25 percent, the result can be devastating. It can increase the potential for congenital abnormalities. The good news is that with regular ultrasounds, this problem can be detected.

g) Labor and birth complications

Twin pregnancies increase the chances of complications. For starters, twin births are often four weeks shorter than single births. Nearly 60 percent of twins are born prior to a standard 36-week term.

h) Premature births

When twins are born early, it almost always means that they will be lighter than what is considered normal for newborns. So most of the time, twin babies are smaller babies than in single pregnancies.

Babies who are born and weigh less than 5.5 lbs (2 kg 494.76g) are more at risk of developing longer term complications, such as: vision loss, hearing loss, cerebral palsy and mental retardation.

There are factors that will increase your propensity to have a premature birth, but some are preventable:

- Being very overweight
- Taking drugs
- Existing health conditions
- Drinking alcohol
- Smoking
- Family history of premature labour
- In vitro fertilization pregnancy

Symptoms that you will have a premature birth are a little harder to discern, since many of them are also common to regular births:

- Lower back ache
- Contractions every 10 minutes or more

- Cramping, gas pains and possibly diarrhoea
- Cramping in the lower abdomen
- Pelvic pressure
- Increased vaginal discharge
- Leaky vagina - fluids
- Flu symptoms

i) Neurological

Twin-to-twin transfusion syndrome (TTTS) is the imbalance of blood between the two little bodies that are sharing one placenta, but have separate amniotic sacs.

Since the placenta is shared, the blood vessels are shared. Sometimes the flow of blood between them becomes unequal, particularly if one is slightly larger. As you can imagine, extra blood is not good for one twin, while less blood flow is not good for the other. Therefore both twins are in danger. Luckily, ultra sounds will help detect this problem.

j) Fetal loss

The loss of one twin while intrauterine is not a common occurrence. However, if it should happen, your physician will know which of the two options will be best for the situation: having a premature birth or leaving the live baby in utero. Either way, the health of the mother and the living baby may not be affected more than temporarily.

k) Cesarean

Many people are concerned that a twin pregnancy generally results in Caesarean births. This is not true for twins, although it may be true for triplets or more. Twins are almost always delivered vaginally.

You'll know the signs:

- If the baby furthest from the cervix is smaller and its head is down, sideways or Breech

- If the baby closest to the cervix is larger and its head is down

- No signs of other complications, such as CPD (cephalopelvic disproportion), when the baby's head is larger than the mother's pelvis.

l) Down Syndrome

Although you will hear talk of Down syndrome among twin births, the odds are actually very slim. According to the UK Down Syndrome Cytogenetic Register, the incidence of Down syndrome among identical twins is about 1-2 in a million. The rate is higher in fraternal twins at 14-15 per million.

These days, you can have tests done to see if your babies have Down syndrome, although the test carries a risk. Speak to your doctor about this. Because of the risk involved, I personally decided not to have the test done.

m) Cerebral Palsy

Cerebral Palsy is more common for multiple births than single births.

n) Mortality Rate

Unfortunately, a big negative about twin pregnancies is that it is more common for babies to be stillborn. However, with these days' technology it happens less and less.

o) Higher chances of complications in labour

With twin pregnancy, there is always that extra chance that things can become complicated during labour. I am not going to list medical terms here and explain what they are. I suggest you research the subject.

p) Higher chances of cot death - get a breathing monitor

Cot death happens and unfortunately the exact causes are still unknown. It is a known fact that cot death is more common with twins and multiple pregnancies. Make sure you it look up or speak to your doctor about what you must do to minimise cot death.

I strongly recommend that you buy a baby respiration monitor, also called a baby breathing monitor.
The respiration monitor I used is called the RM25 respiration monitor and is available here:
www.physicalstate.co.uk. A lot of UK hospitals use it in their baby care unit.

In the UK, you can also get a monitor from
www.lullabytrust.org.uk. The lullaby trust used to be CONI (Care Of Next Infant). This is an organisation that provides support for anyone affected by a sudden infant death or for anyone who had a premature baby. The organisation also advises new parents on the best ways to put a baby to sleep to minimise the risk of cot death. They work closely with the NHS and are present in hospitals and health centres.
Lots of parents use a baby breathing monitor on their baby, just for peace of mind, even if their baby was not born premature (most twins are).

There are lots of similar monitors on the market. For readers outside the UK, I am sorry, as I live in the UK, I cannot recommend a monitor in the USA. Make sure that you investigate very well which monitor is the best one. Remember, usually the cheapest one is not the best one.

You can also have a test to see if your babies have a higher risk of cot death. Talk to your doctor about it.

q) You might not have enough breast milk

Some mums who have a single pregnancy don't produce enough milk to feed one baby. Be prepared, just in case this happens to you, as you need to produce double. I personally breast fed my babies until they were 6 months old, so I was lucky. However, it is good to know that the way breast milk usually works is good for you: the more milk you give, the more your body will produce.

If you are not so lucky to be able to give breast milk for both babies, don't think you are a failure! Millions of babies never get breast milk and they turn out perfectly fine. You can always give breast milk, skip one meal, give breast milk again, skip one meal, etc. Don't get me wrong, you don't actually skip a meal but you give powdered milk instead of breast milk.

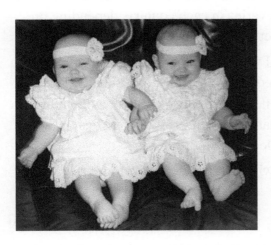

My cuties when they were one year old

r) You might have to rest a lot.

When pregnant with twins, chances are high that you might have to rest a lot after 5 to 6 months into your pregnancy. You need to be prepared in case this happens to you. If you have a job, how is that going to work? Perhaps talk to your boss about it.

My doctor told me at 6 months that I had to rest for the rest of the pregnancy. More specifically, I had to lay down most of the time.

A hospital bed was placed in the middle of our lounge. I have always been an independent businesswoman, so I could run my business from my bed, in the lounge. All I needed was a phone by my side so I could speak to my staff.

s) Extra appointments will be needed

It makes sense that you would need extra appointments once you are pregnant with twins. Undergo them joyfully, because you have succeeded!

If you were having one baby, you could expect to have between five and eight doctor's appointments that are spaced out over your pregnancy. Of course, this varies in each country, depending on how the health system is set up.

With identical twins, you'll want to go for checkups every month, or more, and have more frequent sonograms/ultrasounds. There is always a higher risk of complications when you're having more than one. You'll want to watch for twin-to-twin transfusion, where one twin is getting more blood than the other.

With fraternal twins, you will still want to go for more frequent checkups, but likely not as often as with identical twins.

t) Stop smoking

Easier said than done but you ought to stop smoking, best before you are pregnant, but definitely the moment you find out that you are pregnant.

Smoking is not good in any pregnancy but with a twin pregnancy it carries even more risks for your babies to be premature and very small, therefore coming with more health risks.

Chapter 5) Increase your chances of getting pregnant

1) How to increase your chances of pregnancy

THE most important thing to do first is to find out when your most fertile days are.

Although there is no guarantee that any of these techniques will ensure that pregnancy is the result, they have proven to be effective for many women.

Obviously, that is assuming that both you and your partner's visits to the doctor were encouraging and all systems are go.

I'm sure you have probably read or heard about some of these techniques, as they have been around for years. Some of the suggestions may sound a little unusual, but from my perspective, it is worth investigating.

You can test all of them or select the methods that suit your lifestyle and rhythms and see what happens. You can just practice the ones that you believe in or the ones that make most sense to you. That's what I did.

a) Cervical Mucus Monitoring

According to many doctors, this method is the easiest and possibly the most effective. The key is in the thickness of your cervical mucus from your vagina. Out of a one-four rating system, you will check your cervical mucus daily and rate it like this: 1 is dry or damp, 2 is damp, 3 is thick white or yellowish and 4 is transparent and slippery.

Well, as it turns out, according to a study conducted and authored by Dr. Anne Steiner at the University of Carolina at Chapel Hill, women are two to three times more prone to conception when having intercourse with mucus at the 4 level.

The doctor also revealed that those who checked their cervical mucus consistently were even more likely to get pregnant. Note: This study included 331 fertility-checked women between the ages of 30 to 45.

b) Tracking Body Temperature

It's called Basal Body Temperature testing (BBT). It's almost the same as tracking cervical mucus, but instead you are tracking your temperature within minutes of waking up in the morning. The theory is that your temperature changes as your oestrogen increases and decreases during your normal cycle.

This method is inexpensive and easy to accomplish. Go out and buy a basal thermometer, and a means of tracking your daily temperature, such as a tablet, electronic device or paper kept next to your bed so it becomes a daily reminder.
I personally used this method to find out my most fertile days. You can see a picture of my temperature chart later in the book.

Evidently, the other benefit you get from taking your temperature daily at that time of day is it will help indicate when you are pregnant. Your temperature will stay up during the times that you expect it to be down.

The point is, the more you become familiar with your body's rhythms, the easier it will be for you to detect those windows of opportunity you've both been waiting for and to find your most fertile days, during which you need to have a lot of sex to maximise your chances of getting pregnant.

c) Menses Day Counting

Yes, it's the old calendar counting technique that has been around forever. It is not always effective, due to miscalculations, but it has merit if done right. Having intercourse at the right time with this method is a bit trickier.

Here is the low-down on calendar counting. You ovulate 14 days before your period shows up. That starts the count down - on day one of experiencing bleeding.

So as you count through one entire monthly cycle all the way until you have another period, you will have a baseline. Do this for more than a couple of months to double check. Then all you have to do is count backwards 14 days from the first day of your period and you will be able to narrow the best day down to that one special day that will be luckier than others, as your egg will be ready and waiting.

Now, as I said earlier, many women miscalculate, so a great idea would be to start having intercourse about five-six days before the 14th day before the first day of your period.

d) Weight Control

This may sound like a wives tale or another reason the world is telling you to lose weight and eat healthily, but the truth is that nutrition and weight do make a difference in the area of fertility.

Here's why: Oestrogen regulates ovulation, right? When you are too thin or heavy, your oestrogen levels are not at their prime level. Ideally, you want to make sure your body mass index is within a healthy range.

e) Want to calculate your Body Mass Index (BMI)?

It's easy and only takes a minute.

This first calculation method is in pounds versus metric.

1. Weigh yourself in pounds
2. Measure your height in inches
3. Take the height number and times it by itself
4. Then divide that number by your weight
5. Multiply by the conversion factor of 703

This second method is in metric measurements:

1. Weigh yourself in kilograms
2. Measure your height in meters
3. Times your height by itself
4. Then divide that number by your weight

Here's what it means. You are:

- Underweight if your BMI is less than 19
- A healthy weight if your BMI is within 19 to 24.9
- Overweight BMI is between 25 and 29.9
- Obese is when your BMI is 30 or higher

Now you know whether your weight might have any influence at all on your chances of getting pregnant. Too thin or too heavy are both causes for irregular oestrogen levels.

If you want to get pregnant as badly as I did, then it might be time to do something about any unwanted weight. This is not the best time for any stubbornness, if you're really as serious as I think you are.

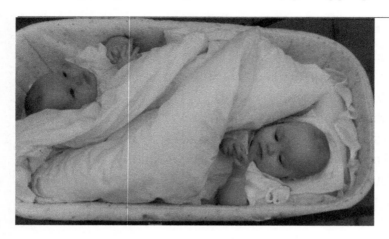

For a long time, because my babies were small when born, I could drive around with two babies in one pram! Very handy!

2) How clothing affects men and women

This attire may not make a fashion statement, but it will enhance your chances to conceive. This might strike you as odd, but listen to the theory behind it. Wearing pink or red elevates your chances for conception.

Why? It may have all started when women, centuries ago, wore these colours when they were having their period. This evidently continued and has been thought to be a subconscious influence. It has become a conscious choice of the colour clothing for some women who want to increase their chances to get pregnant.

- A small series of studies that were published in Psychological Science demonstrated that men were more attracted to women wearing those colours versus other colours.

- The studies also showed that a higher percentage (40 percent) of women who were wearing pink and red were having their period at that time versus the very small percent (7 percent) wearing those colours that were not.

Loose Clothing

Add loose clothing to that mix and you'll have a sexy wardrobe comprised of red and pink loose and comfortable clothes. Of course, your man just needs to stick to the loose part and leave the red and pink to you.

3) Regular exercise

This is one of the few guidelines that can be done too much or too little. The rule of thumb on exercise for increasing fertility is to develop a consistent plan that you can stick to. The best exercise routine will include some type of cardiovascular activity, like walking, light jogging, swimming, cycling or rowing. Thirty to forty minutes a day will make an ample plan.

The goal is to use exercise to help maintain regular ovulation and hormone levels.

For women, cardiovascular routines will help the blood to circulate through the parts of the body that count.

Men might best select exercise activities that don't heat up their reproductive organs. Consider weight lifting, swimming and walking as possibilities.

4) Sleep and relaxation

Getting a good night's sleep is crucial to increasing a man's sperm count and volume. Those men and women who have a difficult time sleeping soundly have a difficult time reproducing.

That's why relaxation is also important. Activities that avoid stress will reduce sleepless nights.

If chronic sleeplessness is an issue, consider taking a yoga or meditation class. These days, you can download a program or there are even apps that can help.

The bottom line on feeling refreshed and rejuvenated is that your body, and his, will know the difference and respond accordingly.

5) Nutrition and diet

Changing your diet is not a tried and true way of increasing your chances of getting pregnant, but according to everything I have read and experienced, it sure does help. It makes sense that when your body is nourished it glows from healthy nutrients running through your system. You know what it takes to make that happen. As you'll see when I layout my personal program, it isn't that difficult.

Processed foods and other junk food are all a habit, just as replacing some of it with healthy and delicious choices can be. Here are some simple dos and don'ts that will help you and your partner get into the most optimal food groove.

6) His and hers: food to include

Follow this basic list to increase your chances of getting pregnant. As you read this book, remember to note the slight changes that you will want to make to increase your chances of birthing twins in a specific gender. I have added checklists in later chapters to help you remember!

a) **Fish with high concentrations of omega-3s**: Try salmon, anchovies, sardines, smelt, mackerel and shad. If you live in an area where these types of fish aren't readily available, you can purchase omega-3 supplements.

b) **Dairy** - particularly high fat dairy like a glass of whole milk or yogurt (kefir). Low-fat dairy products can actually increase infertility.

c) **Protein Switch** - Consider this, if you switch your animal protein with vegetable protein your chances of ovulatory infertility are reduced by over 50 percent. So skip the bacon and reach for cooked legumes instead.

d) **Bananas** - for the B6 vitamin that can regulate your hormones.

e) **Asparagus** - for it's folic acid, which helps reduce ovulation issues.

f) **Shellfish** - for it's B12 magic, which is known to help strengthen egg fertilization (think oysters).

g) **Eggs** - Vitamin D has been found to be an important element in a higher incidence of fertility.

h) **Almonds_** - for their Vitamin E, which is an antioxidant that protects the health of sperm and egg DNA.

i) **Citrus Fruit** - for the Vitamin C that has shown that sperm count and motility are both improved.

j) **Tofu** - Iron is the mainstay in tofu and insufficient amounts can be disastrous to anyone's health.

k) **Peas** - Zinc is the nutrient in peas that helps balance oestrogen and progesterone.

l) **Oysters** - these are high in zinc and help increase male hormones and sperm.

7) Daily vitamin and mineral supplements

Obviously, if any of the foods containing the listed vitamins are not available, then use vitamin supplements.

In fact, folic acid supplements are on the 'must' list even if you are consuming large amounts of asparagus. Folic acid is really important, especially for the woman. It is known to prevent serious ovulatory complications and failure.

It is said that everything on this list, taken daily, will impact your fertility in a very positive way. *It is the combination of these supplements that create the results.*

Even if you have changed your diet and added all of those wonderful items on the food list, go ahead and do both. What do you have to lose?

a) **Vitamin D** - known for creating and balancing sex hormones.

b) **Vitamin E** - improves sperm health.

c) **Vitamin C** - improves hormone levels and increases fertility in women.

d) **B6** - an excellent hormone regulator (also regulates blood sugars).

e) **B12** - improves sperm quality and production.

f) **Folic Acid** - best known for its ability to prevent abnormalities in the foetus, such as mental health problems, cleft lips etc.

g) **Iron** - low iron levels can mean lack of ovulation (60 percent higher chance of having issues than those with good iron levels).

h) **Selenium** - antioxidant that will protect eggs and sperm, plus helps create sperm.

i) **Zinc** - such an important mineral, balances oestrogen and progesterone, plus increased zinc is known to increase sperm levels and fertility in men.

j) **Lipoic Acid** - an antioxidant that protects the female organs and improves sperm quality and motility.

k) **CoQ10** - this is known to provide energy to all of the cells plus increases motility.

l) **Essential Fatty Acids** - you can get them in salmon and the other fish mentioned, but if you don't eat it regularly, it is best to take daily supplements to regulate hormones, increase ovulation, and increase blood flow and cervical mucus.

m) **Choline** - it's kind of a new one on the list, but this helps to reduce birth defects.

8) Things to avoid

You knew it was coming, and here it is. The list of no-nos. You can't be satisfied with adding good vitamins, foods and nutrients without removing those activities, food and beverages that detract from the entire effort. That would make no sense.

As hard as some things may seem, the reward of having that or those babies will be more than worth it.

a) **Herbal teas and botanical supplements** - you don't need to avoid them completely, just watch how much you are consuming.

b) **No raw fish** - stay away from sushi due to the potential mercury content.

c) **No smoking** - enough said.

d) **No alcohol** - bad for sperm motility.

e) **No dehydration** - drink lots of water to keep cervical and ejaculation fluids thin enough to do their job.

f) **No exposure to harmful cleaning agents** - pesticides, any solvents or toxins that smell really strong are probably not good for you to be around.

g) **No laptops on your man's private areas** - laptops get hot and reduce fertility.

h) **No oral sex** - avoid oral sex given to the female when you are trying to conceive. The reason for this is that saliva kills sperm. Saliva contains bacteria that can kill healthy sperm.

i) **No anal sex** - avoid anal sex during conception attempts. Why? Well, you can't get pregnant that way and you should be keeping all the healthy sperm for your vagina!

j) **No sex toys** - avoid sex toys. The reason for this is because some sex toys are jelly sex toys and they can contain softeners which can alter the environment for healthy sperm. So by using sex toys, you could be killing healthy sperm.

9) Special tips for men to increase fertility

We talked about the foods, vitamins and supplements that both of you can be consuming. We also reviewed the myriad of ways that women can increase their chances of pregnancy.

We haven't specifically addressed the men out there. It's true, there are specific things that men can do to increase their own fertility, sperm count, sperm motility and sexual prowess. That sounds like it's going to be a long list, but it's not.

Gone are the days when people were debating between whether men should wear boxers or briefs to encourage healthy and more numerous sperm.

Research studies have been conducted and have no conclusive evidence on which type of underwear might enhance the program. It seems natural that certain garments might hinder sperm production.

When we were trying to get pregnant, my husband never wore tight underwear or tight trousers.

Here is what most experts say:

a) **Stay away from restrictive clothing** - tight jeans, underwear, swimwear or harness gear, basically everything that is tight around the groin area.

b) **Avoid x-rays** - X-rays are a common sperm killer so avoid them during the procreation period.

c) **Keep laptops off your lap** - keep anything hot off of your lap, it hinders sperm quantity.

d) **Avoid hot tubs and baths** - same thing – an environment that's too hot reduces sperm count and possibly quality.

e) **Stay away from stress** - stress is a killer for so many things, so stay relaxed and calm.

f) **No drugs** - not that we are recommending drug use at any time, but definitely stay away at this particular time.

g) **No masturbating for 48 hours** (as this is unproductive ejaculation) before having sex during prime time for ovulation- the woman's most fertile time.

h) **Plan sex for the morning** - sperm count and concentration may be higher in the morning.

i) **No bathtub sex, sex toys, anal sex or cunnilingus** - make sex interesting, but avoid those things that might reduce sperm count or release sperm in the wrong places during ovulation time.

j) **Watch a sexy movie** - Men produce more testosterone and sperm after a sex film.

k) **Stay inside** - after ejaculating into your partner, stay inside for a few minutes to encourage the fertile environment and after several minutes, withdraw very carefully.

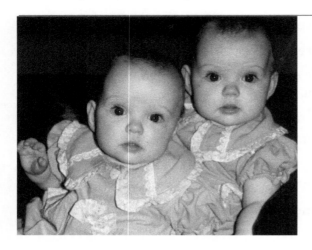

My gorgeous girls just over one year old

10) Female orgasm

Some experts say that the cervical contractions that happen when a woman has an orgasm can pull the sperm up the vagina and closer to the men's egg. During an orgasm, the uterus contracts, causing a vacuum effect that can move the sperm upwards into the uterus.

11) Sex, sex, sex!

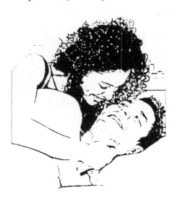

Well, yes I gave this subject a separate header, as I personally believe it has contributed massively to my success in achieving twins. Sex, always sex and lots of sex around your fertile days, that's the message to remember. Just as much as you humanly can! Don't forget to have sex in one of the most fertile sexual positions, discussed in the next section.

Never thought there was a right or wrong way?

In reality, pregnancies happen under all circumstances. Here are a few tips that come from parents who have succeeded and from a few experts.

These tips are just as integral to the program as the other categories I mentioned on earlier pages. So take heed and read up before you engage in what might be your most sexual period since the beginning of your relationship.

For starters, have lots and lots of sex during your fertile days, around ovulation. You now know which times of the month to increase sexual activity in the hopes you hit that one 24-hour period when conditions are perfect. We also recommended starting a week or so before that special day, so it's pretty clear you're going to need to increase your sexual activity, particularly during that time period.

- Using lubricants will probably be necessary, once in a while, due to the increased friction, but here's the thing - if you use too much, it will be counterproductive. More about which lubricants are best to use later in the book, as some lubricants are know to kill healthy sperm.

- Passionate orgasms often deepen the intercourse and increase the chances for conception.

As with anything, the more you do it, the greater chances of success.

12) Best sexual positions

There is no scientific research to prove there are better sexual positions to encourage conception than others. Regardless, common sense tells us that the deepest penetration might be the most potent.

Use sexual positions that encourage the natural tilt of the vagina towards the cervix and positions that assist gravity so the sperm can get quicker/easier to the egg.

Whether you're a believer or not, it surely wouldn't hurt to try each position on ovulation day and see what happens. Or, keep doing what feels the best, as that is extremely important due to the increased sexual activity you will be having.

a) The Missionary Position

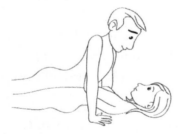

The classic position and most likely the one we were in when we had our first sexual encounter. Everyone knows the man on top position and although it sounds a little dull, if you're creative you can make any sexual position sound interesting, right?

When a woman is lying down on her back, her vagina is tilted towards the cervix. This helps the sperm to swim to the eggs. The woman can also put a pillow under her hip for extra elevation.

b) Doggy Style (Hands and Knees)

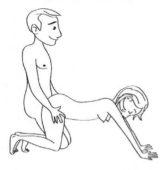

Also called Rear Entry Style. This position creates deep penetration as the woman is on her hands and knees with the man behind. When the man ejaculates into the woman's vagina this way, the sperm can get close to the cervix. His ability to thrust more deeply is enhanced by the leverage of the position.

The other benefit in this position is that the woman's uterus is tipped again.

c) The Rock 'n' Roller.

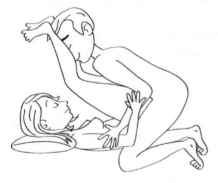

The woman lies on her back with her legs up in the air. The man kneels over her and holds her into the position by bringing his body in front of her and holding onto her. The man keeps the woman up this way. This is a really good position for deep penetration. Ideally, you both stay in this position after ejaculation for at least 20 minutes. The man can't do much other than keep the woman up.

d) The Magic Mountain

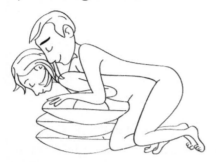

Similar to the Doggy Style position, but with cushions beneath the woman's abdomen - which is actually a little more comfortable for her. The man's legs are spread outside of the woman's for an ideal thrusting position that will provide deep penetration.

In this position, the man kneels behind the woman, whilst she is laying on the pillows, with his legs on the outside of her legs.

It is best to do this position with hardly any cushions, as when the woman bends down, her cervix will be tilted in the right position.

e) The tilt

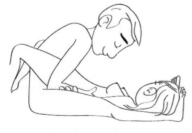

The woman tilts her vagina upwards. The man sits between the woman's legs, with his legs open and the man lifts the woman's hips and supports her in that position. This is a good position for deep penetration. Tilting the vagina towards her cervix is a good way of increasing your chances of getting pregnant.

f) The Dolphin

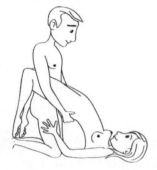

This one does require some effort but this position gives maximum tilting. It is an advanced version of the tilt.

The woman has to put her hips upwards and support herself on her shoulders.

The man helps to support her whilst he penetrates.

Don't forget to stay in this position for 20 minutes after ejaculation! Only joking! You don't want to injure your neck.

g) The Zen Pause

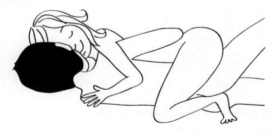

Both man and woman lay on their side and your legs across each other. Press your chests again each other.

h) The Butterfly

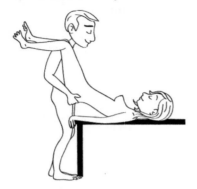

With this position you get really good penetration and tilting. The woman lays on her back and the man in front of the woman. The woman puts her legs over his shoulders and lifts up her hips by holding on to something with her hands. The man holds the woman for support.

This is not an easy one, and best done on a table or a higher surface than the bed. It is worth it though, if you want twins or if you want to get pregnant.

i) The Glowing Triangular.

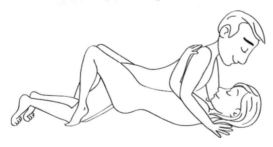

The man is on his hands and knees and the woman lifts up her hips. This way deep penetration is possible. The woman needs to do all the work by pushing her hips up and down whilst the man keeps still.

j) The Plough

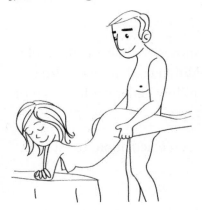

Not an easy one but a good one to strengthen your stomach muscles! The woman is in a position where a really good tilt is possible.

The woman lies on the edge of the bed (or another object), as shown on the picture supporting herself with her elbows. The man stands behind her whilst opening the woman's leg and penetrates into her vagina whilst lifting up the woman's hips.

l) Lap position

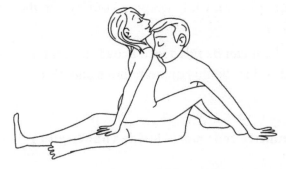

This is a very sexy position for both the woman and man. It's simple to do and most women are familiar with it. The woman sits on the lap of her man and they engage in deep intercourse.

You can sit on the bed or a chair, a table, whatever.

m) Best POST-sex position

Many doctors and sexual specialists subscribe to this method of allowing the sperm to swim for an additional 20 minutes. What this entails is for the woman to put a pillow under her hips to prop them up, allowing a fast path to her uterus.

I personally used to stay in position, after ejaculation, for at least 30 minutes, mostly longer.

13) Attitude and Beliefs

Like with anything, one's attitude has a lot to do with how easily things can happen... or not. If you're resistant to trying new things, opening your mind to life's possibilities and making a few changes, then it is likely that these techniques and methods will fail. If you're sceptical and doubting at every turn, there is little chance for success.

Resistance and closed minds breed failure

Being open to life's bigger picture, while keeping your eye on the ball, is the attitude to adopt.

Once the decision is made, it can be full speed ahead- so get on board. Author Ann Bradford made this quote famous and it's one of my favourites:

"Tell the negative committee that meets inside your head to sit down and shut up."

I'll add to that, "Fire them all!"

Feeling unstoppable and excited about the future is a natural state of being, so give yourself the gift of confidence and trust that you will succeed. Believing is a part of the key.

a) Tips for Staying Positive Every Day

- Make time for you.
- Make time for him.
- Daydream about what you want in your future.
- Think about what makes you happy.
- Concentrate on the upside of everything in your life.
- Journal your thoughts, but be sure not to start a personal pity party.
- Do whatever makes you feel good about yourself.
- Eliminate naysayers and other negative elements or people who bring you down.

When I used to tell my friends how I was planning to have twins, they didn't believe me and said: " Yeah, yeah, we will see". I always replied: "Yes, you WILL see".

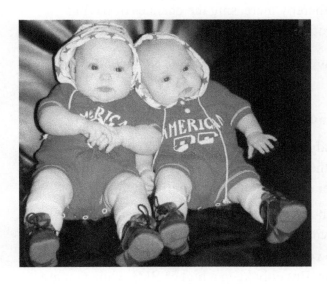

My cuties with their American outfit on!

Chapter 6) Increase your chances of having twins

Factors that will influence your chances of having twins:

a) Your family's history of twins

If twins run in your family, you could be in luck. Heredity could be in your corner as some women have a gene that is inherited for hyper-ovulation. This increases the chance of having multiple eggs being fertilized, and thus having twins. So yes, heredity is a big plus.

Hyper-ovulation means the tendency to release more than one egg during ovulation, thereby increasing the chances of having fraternal (or dizygotic) twins.

Remember that having identical twins does NOT run in your family.

b) Your weight and body size

According to a study by the American College of Obstetrics and Gynaecology, mothers with a Body Mass Index of over 30 had a significantly higher chance of having fraternal twins.

Note: We talked about having a lower BMI to increase your chances of conceiving, in general. The distinction we're making is that if you want to conceive twins, a higher BMI is said to be more advantageous. But only keep a higher BMI while you are trying to conceive, and lower it again once you have succeeded.

As for body size, there is little correlation to body size and increasing the chances of having twins. However, as you can imagine, having wider hips may make it easier for birthing more than one baby. We've added a few yoga poses in a later chapter to help you slowly widen your hip flexors.

c) Have babies when you are older

It is well documented that 17 percent of women over the age of 45 years of age will have twins or multiples. This might be risky, but at least it proves that it is never too late. The only problem with this is that caring for a baby at this age is difficult and having two can be even more challenging at this age and stage of life. I was 33 when I conceived twins.

Although as a woman gets older she is less likely to get pregnant, if she does get pregnant, she is more likely to have twins. The older you are when you are getting pregnant, the more chances you have to have twins.

If you are around 40, you have a 7% more chance to conceive twins. At age 45, that goes up to 17%.

Also, older mothers have an increased risk of miscarriage. Being pregnant, definitely for the first time, when you are older always carries more risks. Luckily, nowadays a pregnancy can be monitored really well and any problems can be detected at an early stage.

d) Have twins once, have twins yet again

If you have had twins once, you are more likely to have them again. Some studies have concluded that having twins once can make it four times more likely of having twins again. The only problem with this is that having two sets of twins can offer even more challenges, despite having the experience.

e) Missing a birth control pill

Inconsistent use of birth control pills can lead to hyper-ovulation and hormonal changes, which can increase the likelihood of having multiples. One way to increase the likelihood of having twins is to try conceiving them when taking the pill sporadically. For being over 99 percent effective, that 1 percent ineffectiveness can be like winning the twin lottery.

A word of warning: taking the pill sporadically is not recommended as your hormones will go "totally up the creek" and might influence the health of your babies. I am only mentioning this method because I came across it during my research. I would personally not use this method of on purpose missing pills.

f) Get pregnant just after you've stopped the pill

The best ways to increase the likelihood of having twins is to try conceiving them just after going off the pill, because your body will undergo hormonal changes and your body will work hard to regulate your hormones. During the first few months after you've stopped the pill, sometimes your ovaries will release 2 eggs.

I stopped taking the pill just before we tried to conceive.

g) Take Folic Acid Supplements

According to Australian research, women who take folic acid when they are trying to conceive have a 40% higher chance of conceiving twins. 40% is a lot! Better start taking the tablets! I did!

I've mentioned folic acid a couple of times, but now that we are talking specifically about increasing your chances of conceiving twins, I'll say it again. This time I'll give it even more emphasis.

It's easy to get more folic acid in the foods you eat, such as: lettuce, spinach, broccoli, asparagus, turnip greens, tomato, strawberries, honeydew melon and even the more unlikely sources of liver and sunflower seeds.

h) Breast feeding while trying to get pregnant again

It is commonly known that you can't get pregnant whilst breastfeeding. Is this so? One study found that women who were breast-feeding were over nine times more likely to have twins when conceiving during this time. Maybe it is the woman's body looking to keep lactating as a means of breast function survival, but this could also be a day care dilemma or a one way ticket to being a stay at home mum.

i) Beverages

A martini or glass of wine might help to get you and your partner in the mood, but alcohol is not great for fertility. Only milk or liquid yogurt (kefir) will increase the chances of having twins. Why? Read on. I recommend no alcohol at all. Get in the mood with a sexy movie instead.

j) Eat Wild Yams

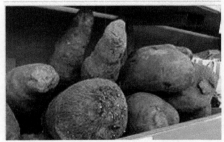

Wild Yams. Source: Wikemedia Commons.

A tribe in West Africa, the Yoruba, has the highest twinning rate in the world, four times above the worldwide average, and a diet high in sweet potatoes (cassava yam) is considered to be the cause. Yam is a type of vegetable. The tribe eats wild yams daily. This tribe and the people of Nigeria have the highest incidence of twins in the world. Perhaps this doesn't work but hey, eating yam has never done anyone any harm so why not try it.

The high levels of certain chemicals in the yam are the reason why more eggs might be released during ovulation.

k) Eat Dairy products

A 2006 study by a doctor at the Long Island Jewish Medical Centre found that a diet high in dairy products raised a woman's chances of having twins. The same study found that vegans had the lowest chances of all. Vegetarians who included dairy in their diet had twins at the same rate as subjects with meat and dairy in their diet.

Dairy products are positively linked to increasing your chances of having twins. According to studies, if you consume dairy products during the time you are trying to conceive, you have 5 times more chance to get pregnant with twins compared to women who avoid dairy products.

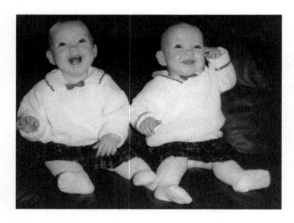

Always happy girls!

l) The Seasons

It seems there could be something to planning to conceive based on the season. While December seems to be the most common month to become pregnant, there are specific months that might be better than others for conceiving twins, which I'll discuss more later.

m) Best time of the month

When you're trying to conceive twins, follow the basic rule of thumb for conception, which is to plan your sex around your most fertile day.

n) Sexual positions

Doctors and medical experts may tell you that there are no better sexual positions than others to increase your chances of having twins. Although that may very well be true, using sexual positions that thrust sperm deep inside the vagina will give you better chances for conception.

o) Frequency of sex

"The more sex, the more chances I have to get twins",

"The more sex, the more chances I have to get twins",

"The more sex, the more chances I have to get twins",

"The more sex, the more chances I have to get twins",

Just walk around thinking this all day and night. That's what I did! I wanted twins so badly so I had a lot of sex! I'm talking 8 to 10 times a day and more. My husband sure used to enjoy those times. You might be thinking - oh boy! Or you might be worried that too much sex will get boring, cause urinary tract infections or any numbers of things. But think about it this way, the more sex you have, the better the odds. And the more sex you have during those high-peak ovulating days, the more you could end up with two little bouncing boys or girls... or one of each!

Just like anything repetitive, you have to find ways to continue to make it interesting enough to want to keep doing it. It is, after all, for a good purpose!

p) Stay in the same position

After ejaculation, the woman should stay in the same position she had sex in for twenty minutes minimum, better even for longer. This is to encourage the swimmers to reach their destination upwards. If you get up immediately and start walking around, gravity will take over and the sperm cells will start going downwards instead of upwards.

q) Sperm-friendly lubricants

The sex and fertility industries have gotten on board and developed quite a few lubricants that don't destroy sperm and might even increase your odds.
Normal lubricants change the pH or acid balance inside the vagina, which affects sperm and reduces the changes of getting pregnant.

Regular lubricants, like KY Jelly, have been known to inhibit sperm and possibly cause DNA damage. There are a couple of brands that are worth noting, as they were actually invented for couples who are trying to conceive. If you can't find them in your local store, they are readily available online.

- **Conceive Plus:** FDA approved and safe for sperm, oocytes (female germ cell involved in reproduction) and embryos. So it's great for having those extra sexy nights and may even help. Sasmar is the only manufacturer that makes a lubricant "that includes calcium and magnesium ions to keep sperm healthy."

- **PreSeed:** This was invented by Dr. Joanna Ellington, who has focused her career on sperm physiology. The company sells a special condom kit that can be used to check fertility. It will catch the semen properly, which others cannot. The lubricant should be applied near the cervix for best results.

- **Yes Baby:** Developed in the U.K., Yes Baby is sperm-friendly and certified organic. Its claims include being vagina friendly, in terms of pH levels.

- **Baby Oil:** If you're on a budget and more inclined to try something that has multi-purposes, then baby oil is your friend. It's inexpensive and works like a charm. It's known to be sperm friendly, although there have been no tests to prove it.

- **Olive Oil** is also suitable.

- **Egg white.** Egg white is also a good lubricant to use. Separate the white from an egg and let it come to room temperature. Salmonella is not a concern here, according to experts, as long as the egg white does not go into one's mouth. Therefore, avoid oral sex.

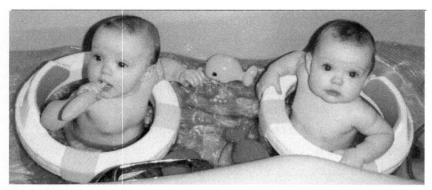

Bath time was always fun!

Chapter 7) Increase your chances of having boys

Both the woman's egg and the man's sperm play a part in determining the sex of the baby.

1) Double the trouble and fun!

If we can increase our chances of having twins and we can increase our chances of having boys, then it makes good sense that we can increase the chances of having twin boys... or twin girls, for that matter.

Not everyone is specific about gender, but many have always dreamed of playing with and mentoring their little boy or girl.

a) More men dream of having boys

In a Gallup poll taken in 2011, the test group of men and women responded with 40 percent stating that they would prefer having boys to girls; 28 percent announced their preference were for girls. The remaining 32 percent had no opinion.

Over the last 70 years, Gallup has conducted similar polls and the results always skewed toward having boys. According to these studies, men were the ones who generally cited the preference for boys, while the women were more apt to state no preference.

It was also revealed that the younger couples in the 18 to 29 age group wanted boys more than girls.

The reasoning for this remains a guess: men want fewer frills and girlie behaviours perhaps.

b) In Eastern Asian countries, boys are always preferred

In Asia, the popularity of boys is mostly due to the fact that boys are more economically capable, as they grow into young men. Women don't have opportunities that result in the higher salaried positions, thus offer less financial stability for their future.

In India and China, the difference is as high as 25 percent more male births than female. That translates to about 100 girls to 125 boys. It boils down to a matter of culture and tradition.

The thing about that is as time goes on, those highly populated countries will have millions of boys who will have little chances of finding wives. A similar thing is happening in India.

c) Twin boys are double the fun

Suffice it to say, if the couple wanted a boy, then having two identical boys would be the utmost in conceptual experiences. Many men around the world feel that having boys will carry on their legacy, while others just want a couple of boys with whom they can play sport.

2) How to increase your chances of having twin boys.

Some of the things I am about to explain might seem contradictory to some of the processes and guidelines that we discussed in earlier chapters.

Remember, this is specifically if you want twin boys. Don't be confused. These recommendations are slight alterations of what you've learned.

This comprehensive list is one I have developed over time from listening to other twin mothers, reading and hours and hours of research.

The first few tips relate to increasing the chances of having twins, in general. The rest pertains to having twin boys. Some of this information is repeated in other chapters in case anyone skips the gender chapters.

a) **Gain Weight:** Believe it. It's been highly suggested that women who have a high BMI have a much better chance of having twin boys.

b) **Eat breakfast:** One study showed a connection between those who ate cereal for breakfast with an increased chance of having boys.

c) **Increase dairy and beef intake:** Because of the growth hormones in cows, it is said to help increase fertility.

d) **Yams:** There might be a connection so it's worth bringing up. There were more twins born in geographic areas where residents consumed more yams. The reason behind this is that there is a chemical in yams that increases ovulation, thus increasing the odds of having twins. If you don't like yams, supplements are available.

e) **The Shettles method:** Shettles is an old-fashioned method for helping to figure out a baby's gender. It's the old XY and XX genetic studies we learned in school. The Shettles method is based on the fact that X sperm are faster but die more quickly and Y sperm are slower but live longer. The way to make this work for you is to have intercourse as close to the ovulation time as possible to allow the faster X sperm get to the egg that is at its nearest point.

f) **Orgasm Delights:** Yes, we said it once and we'll probably say it a few more times in this book. Having orgasms while trying to conceive deepens the chances that the sperm will make it to its destination, due to the contractions of a woman's body during an orgasm. However, you will see later that in order to maximise your choices of having girls, no female orgasm is better.

g) **Alkaline versus Acid Foods:** The vagina is a much more inviting place to male sperm when it is on the alkaline side. Acidity is not an environment for making boys.

h) **Sexual Positions:** Deep penetration will perpetuate the right situation for the sperm to shoot as close to the cervix as possible. You can select your own positions - be as creative as you like. Remember that male sperm are fast swimmers but fast to die off.

i) **Age:** If you're between the ages of 35 and 40, you will have better chances. Some research might show a wider age span, but everything points to twins being conceived at older ages.

j) **Seasons and months:** According to several research studies, the best time to conceive boys is during the summer months.

k) **Have sex close to ovulation:** Some experts believe that if intercourse is closer to the ovulation, the chances are higher to achieve a boy. This is due to the decreased life span of the Y carrying sperm. Aim to have sex often, say about one day before ovulation.

l) **Chinese Birth Chart for Conceiving a Boy:** Many people are believers in the Chinese calendar for predicting births, mortality and fertility. Even if you aren't a believer, it's pretty interesting. The chart will show you at which age and month you would be more likely to conceive boys.

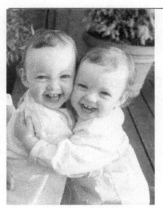

My favourite picture ever! That's why it is on the front cover.

Chinese Birth Chart for Conceiving Boys

Conception Months	Mother's Age at Time of Conception
January	19, 21, 23, 24, 26, 28, 30, 31, 32, 34, 35, 37, 39, 41, 43, 44
February	18, 20, 22, 23, 25, 27, 29, 33, 35, 36, 38, 40, 42, 44, 45
March	19, 22, 24, 25, 26, 28, 31, 32, 33, 34, 36, 37, 39, 41, 43, 45
April	18, 20, 23, 24, 27, 33, 35, 37, 38, 40, 42, 44
May	18, 20, 22, 23, 29, 36, 38, 39, 41, 43, 44
June	18, 19, 20, 23, 24, 25, 26, 29, 37, 40, 42, 44
July	18, 19, 20, 23, 24, 27, 28, 29, 38, 40, 41, 43, 45
August	18, 19, 20, 22, 25, 26, 27, 28, 29, 33, 35, 37, 39, 41, 42, 44
September	18, 19, 20, 23, 25, 27, 28, 29, 36, 38, 40, 42, 43, 45
October	18, 19, 23, 25, 27, 28, 36, 37, 39, 41, 43, 44
November	18, 20, 23, 25, 30, 34, 35, 36, 38, 40, 42, 43, 45
December	18, 20, 25, 27, 30, 31, 32, 33, 34, 35, 36, 37, 41, 43, 45

Chapter 8) Increase your chances of having girls

1) Identical twin girls

As we pointed out, some people have a longing to have boys and some just can't get their minds off of having twin girls.

Interesting to note, girl twins have fewer physical problems than boy twins, who have lower than average birth weights and more respiratory and neurological problems. In general, fraternal twins or girl twins are known to be healthier and have fewer pre-term deliveries than twin boys.

The timing for getting pregnant may be a little more difficult for a girl than a boy. Remember the Shettles method? We talked about how X sperm are fast but die sooner, and Y sperm are slower but live longer?

Well, in that example we showed how having sex closer to the actual day of ovulation would work the best. The travelling egg would be at its closest so the X sperm could work its magic and penetrate the egg to produce a boy.

Well, if you want to conceive girl twins, you will need to time everything differently. These tips will help you to plan intercourse for a girl.

a) **Timing of sex:** To have twin girls, you will want to time your intercourse so that it is several days before ovulation. Remember, if you have intercourse too close to ovulation, your chances of having boys is greater. The sperm with the X chromosome have a longer life span than the male sperm, therefore intercourse that takes place early might increase your chances of having a girl. So you must have sex no closer than 4 days before your ovulation. This way, the Y chromosome, or man's sperm, is likely to be expired and the X carrying sperm is still OK. The X carrying sperm will be in the fallopian tube waiting. If an X chromosome fertilises the egg, a girl will be conceived.

b) **Sexual positions:** Unlike the deep penetration positions we have mentioned in earlier chapters, you will want to use positions that are shallower to let the Y sperm reach the egg later in its process. Some say the missionary position is best, but I think you can figure out which works best for you, as it may depend on penis size and length and the man's thrusting style.

c) **Fewer orgasms:** It is really the opposite of what we have previously discussed and will make sense. Just as we told you that orgasms can deepen the penetration and potential for sperm making it to their destination, fewer orgasms will give the Y sperm a better chance of surviving all the way to the egg, while the X sperm die off.

d) **The Whelan Method:** Dr. Whelan's technique is said to produce a 57 percent success rate on conceiving girls. Her theory includes having sex two to three days before ovulation.

Neither the Shettles method nor the Whelan method are scientifically proven, as there has not been a great deal of research done to substantiate the claims.

e) **Change your pH:** You will want your body's internal environment to be more acidic than alkaline. Eat foods that remain acidic once they are in the body. Good health generally relies on a pH that is more alkaline than acidic, but for the purpose of having twin girls try to change it with the foods you eat. The thing to note is that an acidic pH will prohibit the body's ability to absorb all of those minerals and nutrients, so keep that in mind.

Be careful though, a body too acidic is not a great place to stay, so be judicious about when and how much you partake. Try for a few days (3-4) before ovulation. Some acid producing foods are: white flour, eggs, dairy, meat, coffee, sodas and artificial sweeteners.

f) **Avoid highly alkaline foods:** This recommendation, as with most of the special food enhancements and restrictions, is meant as the diet to use a few days prior to having intercourse for conception. So the foods you will want to avoid will be: apples, almonds, lemons and mushrooms. There are a couple sources in the last chapter that will provide complete lists.

g) **Lower salt intake:** Although there may be no proof to support this, a diet lower in salt is healthier anyway. In addition, it is said to increase your chances of having girls. It would be a great time to cut out chips, fries, processed foods that are high in sodium, olives, salty meats and to reduce the amount you use in cooking. If you must, consider using a pinch of sea salt, which is healthier.

h) **Lower potassium intake:** Potassium, which is found in bananas, creates a comfortable environment for male sperm, so it makes good sense to avoid foods that contain it. Potassium is found in: potatoes, spinach, Swiss chard, beans, winter squash, dates, yogurt, avocado, tomato sauce and paste, fish (salmon and clams), raisins, dried apricots and cantaloupe.

i) **Eat more fruit and vegetables:** Following on from the potassium note above, avoid the foods on that list and opt for more broccoli, celery, peas, cauliflower, berries and also foods that are high in calcium and magnesium.

j) **Drink milk and runny yoghurts.** I did this when I tried to get pregnant with girls so basically I don't care if other people say it doesn't work, as it worked for me.

k) **Hot bath or hot tub:** Heat seems to reduce the male sperm count, so it makes sense that a hot bath prior to having sex would be a smart course of action to increase your chances of having girls.

As a contradiction to this, my husband did NOT take hot baths. The reason behind that decision is because we didn't even know if my husband could produce healthy sperm, as he had a reverse vasectomy just before we started trying to conceive. So we also had to focus on trying to get pregnant in the first place combined with trying to get identical twin girls, in order to achieve my dream.

2) Wives Tales with little substance

There are so many wives tales that have been passed down over the years, so it is difficult to address all of them. But some sound so real. I thought it might be a great time for a review. Plus, one never knows - right?

- **Baby's heart rate**: It has been said that if a baby's heart rate is above 140 bpm (beats per minute), the baby will be a girl. If it is under 140 bpm, it will be a boy.

- **Belly shape:** If you have a big round belly that is high, you're having girls. If you have a smaller belly, you're having boys.

- **Ring test:** This one is a bit funny. Put your wedding ring on a string and tie it. Then hang the ring over your belly. If it circles, it's a boy. If it goes back and forth instead, it is a girl.

- **Mom's face shape:** Another somewhat amusing tale - if the mother's face gets more full while pregnant, she is having a girl. If it begins to look narrow and more elongated, it is a boy. I know my face got more full when I was pregnant. A lot more full!

- **Acne:** It is said that if the mother has acne while pregnant, she will have a girl. If not, it will be a boy.

- **Mayan tale:** Add the mother's age and the year of conception together. If the sum is an odd number, the babies will be boys. If the sum is even, they will be girls.

- **Garlic:** Not sure you will want to try this, but if the mother eats cloves of garlic and her skin doesn't smell like garlic - it will be girls. If she smells like garlic - bingo - boys!

- **Legs:** If the mother's legs get really big, she's having boys. If the legs stay their normal size, girls will be in your future.

- **Bread:** Mother's who eat the ends of the loaves of bread are destined to have boys, while those who eat the middle will have girls. For your information: I never eat the ends of bread, only the middle.

- **Clumsy:** Graceful actions by the mother mean she is having a girl and clumsy means boys. Well, that one might be true, right ladies?

- **Water:** Drinking water and staying hydrated is so important for a healthy pregnancy. It is said that if the mother doesn't drink enough water, her babies will have dirty amniotic fluid. Rest assured - this is not true.

3) Chinese birth chart

Since we showed you the Chinese calendar that may improve your chances of having boys, we want to give you the same benefit of checking your age against the months to see the ones that might be conducive for having girls. Again, the claims have almost 90 percent accuracy and success rate - so perhaps there is something to the Chinese ability to predict birth and death.

The chart is used for women between the ages of 18 and 45 and although it pertains to singleton births as well as twin births, the possibility of its authenticity is pretty high, according to everything I've read and heard.

After all, the Chinese are known for having ancient mysteries that are founded by seeing the results. Chinese medicine and treatments are being studied by the western medicine industry more than ever before for their efficacy.

Finally, western physicians are seeing the value in their eastern counterparts' claims and giving credence to the possibilities enough to dabble and learn.

Chinese Birth Chart for Conceiving Girls

Conception Months	Mother's Age at Time of Conception
January	18, 20, 22, 25, 27, 29, 33, 36, 38, 40, 42, 45
February	19, 21, 24, 26, 28, 30 31, 32, 34, 37, 39, 41, 43
March	18, 20, 21, 23, 27, 29, 30, 35, 38, 40, 42, 44
April	19, 21, 22, 25, 26, 28, 29, 30, 31, 32, 34, 36, 41, 43, 45
May	19, 21, 24, 25, 26, 27, 28, 30, 31, 32, 33, 34, 35, 37, 41, 42, 45
June	21, 22, 23, 27, 28, 30, 31, 32, 33, 34, 35, 36, 38, 39, 41, 43, 45
July	21, 22, 25, 26, 30, 31, 32, 33, 34, 35, 36, 37, 39, 42, 44
August	21, 23, 24, 30, 31, 32, 34, 36, 38, 40, 43, 45
September	21, 22, 24, 26, 30, 31, 32, 33, 34, 35, 37, 39, 41, 44
October	20, 21, 22, 24, 26, 29, 30, 31, 32, 33, 34, 35, 38, 40, 42, 45
November	19, 21, 22, 24, 26, 27, 28, 29, 31, 32, 33, 37, 39, 41, 44
December	19, 21, 22, 23, 24, 26, 28, 29, 38, 39, 40, 42, 44

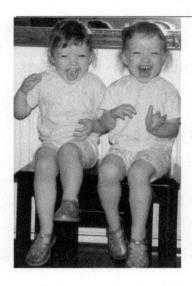

My girls were ALWAYS having fun, giggling together. As you can see from this picture, it wasn't always giggling, it was more like laughing their heads off!

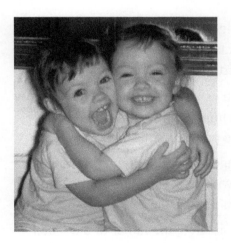

Hugs and kisses were a regular scene in our house!

Chapter 9) Alternate methods to having twins

Special Twin Methods - Fertility Drugs

During the last few decades, additional options for enhancing conception have become very popular. Drug-induced fertilization, medications and even holistic methods have come to the forefront. Many of the new methods began producing frequent multiple births, yet sometimes creating severe traumas to the mother's body.

Personally, I'm all for doing things naturally. But I realize that there are many fertility-challenged couples out there so thank goodness these options are available.

a) In Vitro Fertilization (IVF)

In vitro fertilization is definitely going to give you higher chances of conceiving and producing twins. Statistically, this is a fact. Yet, only about 5 percent of infertile couples use this method.

Taking a step back, I will explain exactly what in vitro is and how it is used. The first step includes injecting hormones into the mother so additional eggs will be produced during her cycle.

Once the eggs are at the right stage of development, they are removed and placed into a dish with a special fluid. The timing of this is crucial and possibly why it often fails.

After the eggs are collected and situated, the father or a donor's sperm is collected and mixed into the dish with the eggs in the hope that fertilization will take place.

Once the egg is fertilized, after about 5 days, it is transferred into the woman's uterus in the hope that her body will accept the pregnancy.

The method is simple, but not always fool proof. In fact, it may require repetition, which can be costly.

About 25-30 percent of women who use in vitro fertilization will have twins. This might be one of the more costly ways of trying to have twins, but the percentages are pretty impressive.

Advantageous:
- For couples who are carriers for certain disease traits, as the sperm or egg can come from a donor.
- For couples who want multiple births.
- Women and/or men who have infertility issues.

Disadvantages:
- Multiple births are likely and twins are not guaranteed.
- You could end up with triplets or more.
- In vitro is very expensive so if it has to be repeated, it can add up.
- The average cost is close to $13,000 / £8,000 per treatment. This obviously can vary in each country.
- It is a fairly invasive procedure.

b) What is Clomid?

Clomid, also called Clomiphene, is an oral ovulation prescription that can greatly increase the chances of having twins. The only problem is that having more than just twins is also more likely, as the ovaries drop more eggs in each cycle. Other drugs such as Gonadotropin and hormone shots can also stimulate ovulation and increase the likelihood of the ovaries releasing more eggs.

Advantages

- It's one of the most successful methods for increasing the chances of pregnancy, even among those who don't have fertility issues.
- Proven to increase the production of eggs.

Disadvantages

- Same as in vitro -the chances of multiple births is high.
- Blurry vision or floaters during treatment may occur.
- Allergic reactions are possible.
- Lower abdomen swelling is possible.
- Potential weight gain can occur.

c) Acupuncture

This new age treatment has been around for about five centuries (5,000 years old) and has been known to heal many ailments, including infertility.

Acupuncture is based on the theory that your body might have blocked qi (pronounced chi), which is the energy that flows through your body.

In a study carried out in 2002 by a group of German researchers, acupuncture treatments enhanced conception in 160 women who were also using IVF treatments. The results showed that there were increased pregnancies among those who had undergone the acupuncture treatments.

Since it is also known as a treatment that induces relaxation, this could be partly the reason for its success in the test group.

The bottom line is if you want to try acupuncture, be sure to find a practitioner who has worked with couples or women who are trying to conceive.

d) Yoga can help fertility and birthing

We've talked about how reducing stress can help conception, so it won't surprise you that yoga poses might be something to consider. If you know anything about yoga, you're aware of its stress-relieving results. So that benefit is a given - it will keep you calm and alert.

There are many who subscribe to specific yoga poses for affecting fertility by increasing the blood flow to specific areas of the body- like the pelvis.

Additionally, all of the yoga poses offer the benefit of keeping the mother's body limber, which will help during the birthing process.

There is no point showing you pictures of the yoga poses as, if you are planning to do yoga, you will soon find out how to do the different poses. Different poses have different names and I am not a yoga person myself. I suggest you search online to find a picture of the yoga poses listed here.

Potentially fertility-boosting poses:

<u>Half Ankle to Knee pose</u>

This will help open up your hips and align your uterus, if done properly.

How to do it:

- Sit with your legs extended and a straight back.
- Flex the right foot and press the left hand's palm against its sole.
- Simultaneously, press the right hand against the knee and gently press it down.

- Gently stretch the knee up and down so it relaxes the hip joint.

Bridge pose

A great sexual position as well, the Bridge pose will help connect your centre: hips, pelvis and lower back. It will help your endocrine and immune systems.

How to do it:

- Lay on your back with your legs in a 90-degree angle.

- Slowly lift up the buttocks, while tightening everything in the mid-centre.

- Arms are flat against the ground with palms up.

- Use the strength of the arms for more leverage.

Side lunge

This pose is another great way to increase the flexibility of the hips and pelvis. You may have learned this in another type of exercise class. The most important thing is that your knee is never over the ankle; it should remain at a 90-degree angle.

How to do it:

- Step into a wide lunge with your knee bent and hips square to the front. Be mindful of the hips, as they tend to turn slightly when remaining in this pose for long.

- Bend the back knee slightly while pulling in your tailbone, tucking in the pelvis.

- Raise the opposite arm of the front-extended leg up into a nice stretch.

- Repeat on the opposite side. Always repeat one-sided poses on both sides.

Yogini Squat

This helps create a strong centre and again adds a great deal of flexibility to the pelvis area. All of these pelvic poses will be great for your increased sex life too!

How to do it:

- Squat comfortably, making sure your knees are wider than your hips.

- Put the palms of your hands together and your elbows apart.

- Using your elbows, put pressure on both knees to slightly move them further apart.

- Sit as straight as you can during this pose and hold for as long as you are comfortable.

Goddess Pose

This pose will help to open your pelvis and hips and is very relaxing, which will be very important during the entire term.

How to do it:

- Lying on your back, bend your knees and let them fall loosely to each side of your body.

- Place the bottoms of your feet together.

- With your hands on your belly, breathe slowly and focus on relaxing while you continue for 3 to 5 minutes.

- If you're not at the flexibility level that allows a comfortable stretch for your legs, you can put pillows or rolled towels under each knee. If you repeat this daily, you will continue to stretch out the pelvis and reduce any discomfort.

Breathing and Relaxation Pose

This should come at the end of your yoga practice and can be used at any time you are feeling stressed or uptight.

How to do it:

- Lie on your back with your legs comfortably situated without strain. Put your arms alongside your body, with palms up and eyes gently closed. Make sure your mouth is also in a loose and relaxed position.

- Breathe in, starting from your lower belly and moving up to the lungs. Hold for the count of ten.

- Breathe out slowly through your mouth in a very controlled manner. Repeat for five to ten minutes.

In all yoga poses, remember to breathe deeply and concentrate on each muscle group. If you feel pain or too much pressure, back off a little, but also continue to breathe into the pain or pressure.

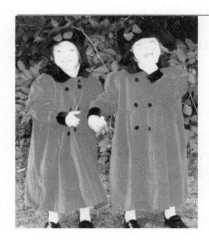

My smart looking girls at 4 years old.

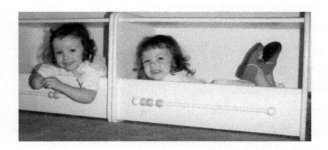

Chucking out all the toys and getting in the toy box themselves!

Chapter 10) Planning your checklist

I've organized it for you

These checklists will come in handy when you want to get serious about planning and preparing for conceiving and birthing twins. Use the lists to trigger yourself and partner to get proactive and start making the changes that can make the difference between having twins or not.

1) One year planning

Create a month-by-month plan to make it simple by reviewing the following elements;

- ✓ Are you in a decent financial position to handle the costs of twins? Make a list of necessities and associated costs.
- ✓ Decide if you want to gain a little weight.
- ✓ Determine your BMI.
- ✓ Review your current diet.
- ✓ Start tracking your ovulation.
- ✓ Ladies: a trip to the Doctor.
- ✓ Men: a trip to the Urologist.
- ✓ Review your wardrobes - make sure loose fitting clothing is a large part of your casual clothing.
- ✓ Review current exercise regimens.
- ✓ Improve sleep habits.
- ✓ Begin using daily vitamins and minerals.

2) Nine months before *really* going for it!

- ✓ Cervical Mucus Monitoring.
- ✓ Check your BMI.
- ✓ Start altering your diet, if you haven't already.
- ✓ Ladies: enjoy wearing pink and red.

- ✓ Start tracking your ovulation.
- ✓ Ladies: a trip to the Doctor.
- ✓ Men: a trip to the Urologist.
- ✓ Increase dairy and milk intake.
- ✓ Switch protein source to mostly vegetables.
- ✓ Start eating yams frequently.
- ✓ Include all foods already suggested in this book in your diets.
- ✓ Continue taking vitamins and minerals.
- ✓ Make sure to be consuming or taking Omega 3.
- ✓ If you haven't already, stop smoking, eating sushi and drinking herbal teas and botanical supplements.
- ✓ Time to reduce or eliminate alcohol intake.
- ✓ During off-work hours, wear comfortable, loose clothing.
- ✓ Start gathering sexual paraphernalia: adult movies, lubricant and anything else that will keep things interesting instead of making sex something that stops being fun.
- ✓ Ladies: If you haven't already, start your cardiovascular routine for about 30 minutes a day.
- ✓ Men: Same goes for you - if you haven't selected your workout, weight training is a great start.
- ✓ Have you determined whether you want to try for twin girls, twin boys, fraternal or whatever happens? Now would be a good time to do that.
- ✓ Time to give up those hot Jacuzzis.
- ✓ Men: Be attentive to putting warm things around your groin area, like laptops.
- ✓ Stop smoking and/or taking any drugs if you haven't already.
- ✓ Use positive affirmations to replace any doubts.
- ✓ Stay intimate emotionally - a strong connection between partners can help.

3) Six months before

- ✓ Blood pressure check.
- ✓ Create your fertility calendar.
- ✓ Practice best sexual positions and orgasms.
- ✓ Attitude check - focus on your conception goals.
- ✓ Have you weighed in on the risks? Prepared?
- ✓ Have you determined what months are best for conception based on the twin gender you want. Now is the time to plan and incorporate the specific changes in the routine.
- ✓ Pay particular attention to your diet.
- ✓ Continue eating the new foods on the list to get all of your vitamins and minerals naturally.
- ✓ The foods and habits you have eliminated will be good for so many things - but most importantly -they will encourage a fertile environment for twin conception.
- ✓ Have your ovulation calendar as perfected as possible - hopefully you have been keeping track.
- ✓ Consider how you would handle twin feedings, naps, breast-feeding, formula and look at the cold reality of the work involved for about three years.
- ✓ Are you saving money? In the event you have twins you want to be ready, financially.
- ✓ Thinking about how you will feel when you have those little dolls. What could be more precious than two tiny little bodies that are psychologically connected?
- ✓ If you believe in it, try planning for conceiving during the months indicated on the Chinese calendar.
- ✓ Practice your sexual positions and different techniques to keep it all sexy and fun. You can expect to feel a little bored at times, but with the right preparation, you'll be able to meet the challenge!

✓ Now is the best time to increase your intake of folic acid. It wouldn't hurt to take an oral supplement in addition to eating from the list of foods listed below. Not only will these give you extra folic acid, you'll be getting a bundle of your necessary vitamins. Remember, folic acid can help increase the chances of conception plus decrease the chances of abnormalities in twin pregnancies. We want our twins to be the healthy!

Foods with Folic Acid:

- Fortified cereals and grains

- Cooked lentils

- Spinach

- Broccoli

- Sunflower seeds

- Beans

- *Asparagus*

- Enriched pasta

- Cantaloupe

- Egg yolk

- Liver

- Tomatoes

- Turnip greens

- Lettuce

- ✓ Limit caffeine (although there are two schools of thought on the matter).
- ✓ Determine whether you are at your ideal BMI.
- ✓ Start doing some of the activities that you won't be able to do for a while. Things as simple as going to the movies to see something you'll enjoy. Once you're pregnant, you'll be too pooped to do some of the things you're taking for granted right now.
- ✓ Stash a secret twin fund somewhere in the house and start saving on top of your other savings. Not trying to scare you, but you'll use all the money you have during the first couple of years... and beyond, if you're planning higher education for your twins.

4) Three months before

- ✓ Sleep, sleep, sleep.
- ✓ Use your fertility calendar to plan your sexual escapades. Can't stress enough how important it is to keep things interesting.
- ✓ Visualize what it will be like to have two infants and then toddlers underfoot. Think of the joys that you will feel and the amazing connection you will witness.
- ✓ Take photos of your life as you know it, because you won't remember it afterwards.
- ✓ In fact, you will want to make sure you have a good tablet or phone with a camera and video capability. You're going to want to record all of the things that are about to transpire if all goes well.
- ✓ Have you considered your current living space and how long it will be sufficient for an expanded family? You probably have a few years before you need to concern yourself with that, but if you live in an NYC or Paris studio flat, you will want to have a plan.

- ✓ Consider how the job situation will change. Will one of you have to stay at home? Perhaps you will have to lie down for a big part of the pregnancy.
- ✓ Make a dental appointment. Current research links oral health to overall health, similar to other mammals. Women with gum disease have a higher incidence of miscarriages.
- ✓ Take your last bit of independent travel with friends, your partner or family! It's going to be a while until you can do that again. Honestly.
- ✓ Consider letting your hair go au natural. Do you want to be dying your hair during pregnancy? It's your call.
- ✓ Get your sex on again. Follow your calendar and make it happen.
- ✓ Talk to your loved one about how you might raise the tiny tots. Twins can be a handful, especially when they know they have you wrapped around their fingers.

5) One month before

- ✓ Continue all of your new habits - don't miss a beat.
- ✓ Get even friskier in the bedroom - pull out all the stops.
- ✓ Make a list of things you'll need after you become pregnant.
- ✓ Expect to become pregnant with twins - visualize.
- ✓ Find new ways to eat some of the foods you're not crazy about. If you don't love yams, make mashed yams and russet potatoes. There's always a way.
- ✓ Start thinking of how to decorate the nursery.
- ✓ Realize that patience, confidence and having a strong belief will be great tools.

✓ Start having more frequent sex 8-10 days before the day of ovulation. If you can't make 8 times, I suggest you try for minimum 3 times.

✓ If you haven't used this before, start using the cervical mucus test. It will give you another way to determine when you are most fertile.

✓ Have you thought about if you will breastfeed? If not, how do you plan to feed twins?

✓ Both of you need to stay healthy. It's no time to get a cold, or any ailment for that matter.

✓ Continue your cardiovascular routine of 30 minutes a day while your partner is manning up to some weight lifting.

✓ Menu planning will help incorporate as many of the proactive vitamins and minerals into your daily diet as possible. We have provided a few recipes to get you started.

✓ If you haven't started one yet, start a journal or diary to keep track of all of the efforts. You'll soon see what works!

Sample Menu Planning:

You might want to pre-plan your menus to make sure all of the new diet items are included. Remember to check the suggested changes in diet if you are trying for a specific gender.

- Baked salmon with a side of mashed yams and potatoes.

- Portobello mushrooms stuffed with spinach, shredded cheese, chopped broccoli and mixed rice. Remember, if you want girls, to avoid mushrooms.

- Steamed spinach with lemon and olive oil, sprinkled with a little Parmesan cheese.

- Baked yam topped with peas, kale, plain yogurt, shredded cheese and olives.

- Milk smoothies: Blend up some of your favourite fruits and milk. Add a small amount of honey to taste.

- Yogurt smoothies: Use plain yogurt, spinach, chocolate powder or honey to taste, banana and blend with ice.

- Cheese Fondue: Melt Swiss or other cheeses with a little milk and flour. Heat until blended. Dip part-cooked or raw vegetables into the fondue while still warm. Works best in a fondue pot.

- Stuffed Portobello Mushrooms: Clean mushrooms, cut up the stems. Sauté onions and garlic in butter until soft and transparent. Be sure not to overcook the garlic. Add chopped mushroom stems and spinach. Spoon mixture into the mushrooms. Top with cheese and bake for 15-20 minutes until cheese melts and slightly browns. Some of these mushrooms are large, so you can easily make a meal out of a couple of these per person.

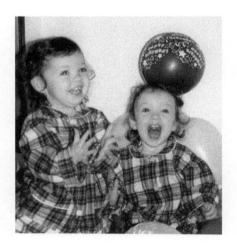

In their pyjamas after their birthday party, giggling, as usual!

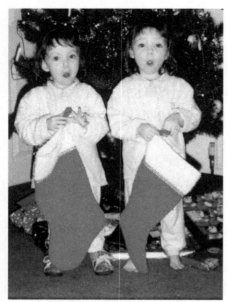

Being silly at Xmas!

Chapter 11) Questions you are likely to have

1) Questions you're likely to have

Well, you did it! You managed to work your own magic after synthesizing all of the information in this book. I am guessing you'll probably take your favourite information and develop your own hybrid plan.

It's anyone's guess which are the most important elements of any plan, or if it's the whole package that makes twins happen.

You probably have lots of questions. I've included a reference section at the end of this book, so you can easily find everything you'll need and more.

I strongly encourage you to join forums, seek twin-special websites, read the comments, ask questions and help one another through the growing pains of twin parenthood.

I am going to cover a few questions I know you'll want answers to immediately:

a) My twins were slightly different sizes when they were born, is this normal?

This is perfectly normal and it is often the case that the first-born twin weighs more than the second one. Generally, the heavier twin is closest to the vaginal opening, due to gravity. But what often happens is one grows a tiny bit faster and ends up being the larger of the two (like my girls). Although there has been little research to substantiate anything conclusive, I think it's interesting to note.

Remember, identical twins are sharing and possibly competing for resources when they are in the womb, so it would be less likely for the two little bodies to progress at the same rate.

b) How can I tell if my twins are identical?

The best way is to have a DNA test after the birth. Another way to know is by examining the placenta after birth. Neither method is fool proof, as doctors have been wrong in their identification of fraternal versus identical twins.

After all, most parents of twins are not seeking physicians or midwives who specialize in twin births. You have to keep that in mind during the entire pregnancy.

You may have gathered more information and talked to more twin parents than the doctor has in his entire career. Even with sonograms, the specialist running the machine is probably not an expert in twin scans.

c) Your body, your twins

That's another reason you're educating yourself. No one can do it for you - but having every piece of information under one roof will give you access to every aspect that will help you navigate the entire process, starting from the idea of having twins all the way through to how to handle two babies.

I suggest that you do your own research, regardless of what any doctor tells you. Your doctor probably never had twins so they don't know everything there is to know. Do your own research at each stage of your pregnancy and talk to other twin mums online.

2) What mothers of twins can expect

Since multiple births have increased, one would think having twins is no big deal - but it is. Carrying two little beings inside one's body is not an everyday occurrence.

During the twin pregnancy, women are at a higher risk of:

- Early delivery (premature births).
- Getting diabetes.
- Gaining additional weight.
- Preeclampsia (rise in blood pressure).

I have already covered these in more detail earlier in this book.

a) Things to expect ahead of time

Well, think about it - you'll have an instant family of four or more, depending on whether you have other children. That's a lot to juggle if you're not used to it.

I won't lie, it's demanding and exhausting - even more than if you had birthed one child, obviously. Of course, all babies are different and you could be lucky with two little ones who love to sleep.

b) It's harder to take turns

When you have one baby, you and your partner can take turns. But with two, it's not quite as easy. If you don't have the luxury of having a family member or nanny to help out in the early hours of the morning, you will both be exhausted. That exhaustion probably won't go away until the twins have settled into their own little schedule.

Being exhausted effects your life in pretty negative ways, so having a strategy ahead of time will be key to survival and enjoyment.

c) Strategy for staying fresh

What you want to do is create a rhythm that works for your body. So, you can't sleep eight hours in a row? Sorry for the tough love, but get over it. You wanted this.

Instead, get in a different habit while you are pregnant. Although pregnancy requires solid rest, you can learn to do it in two-three separate clumps. If you're a sound sleeper when your head hits the pillow, then this strategy can work.

By the time the twins are born, you will have adapted some new sleep behaviours that nearly mimic the babies.

Take every opportunity you can to take a power nap! When your babies are asleep, take a nap yourself.

d) Share duties with a friend

Hopefully you will have met other new mothers and maybe even a few who've had twins. If not, there are several ways to meet up with women and men in the same situation.

If you have a relative handy, that will work also. If not, go onto Craigslist.com or Meetingup.com or check through the forums to see if there are any localized groups who may offer help.

You might create a "Let a Mom Sleep" program, where you each take turns in giving the other a solid block of time to catch up on sleep.
Be creative ahead of time and it will pay off. This period won't last forever.

Like with any children, the work is upfront and begins getting easier after the first few years.

3) Do twins take care of each other?

It's one thing to see two siblings play together, but almost an entirely different experience with twins. Some twins even have their own language, which is termed idioglossia.

As they grow, they will end up entertaining and teaching one another. They may learn things at a faster rate because of it.

Their personalities aren't always similar. Some twins have opposite temperaments and others are as identical as they look. The thing you can almost always count on is that they will be their own closest and best friends for their entire lives.

4) Are twins competitive?

Of course, that depends on the twins. While it is likely that they will spur each other on to excel, there may be times when one is given an accolade and the other isn't. The pressure that is caused is never a good thing when they are little. Think about how you will handle it if one becomes potty trained before the other. Does your praise for one naturally create resentment and envy from the other?

a) Twins are generally their own cheerleaders

However, as they grow older they will have to deal with the real world and competition, success and failure are all part of it. A lot of how they interact with one another as they age will be due to the similarities and differences of how you treat them as infants and toddlers.

b) Do twins stay alike their entire lives?

Of course, that depends on the twins. But I have heard more stories than not of twins remaining innately similar their entire lives. Most remain confidents and best friends forever, also.

c) Can other siblings tell them apart?

Most siblings do have an advantage of getting to know the unique personalities of their twin brothers or sisters. So, yes, they can generally tell them apart.

5) Will my other kids feel jealous?

As with all children, they are going to determine their relationships themselves. But you can certainly set the tone. If you treat the twins like they are more important, then explain to the others why. Twins require a bit more attention for the first few years, particularly if they were born premature.

As the twins age, it is important that you recognize their individuality, just as you do with the others, if you have more. That is the reason why you have to stop dressing them the same, after a few years.

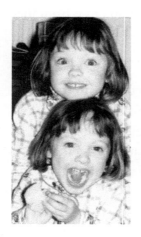
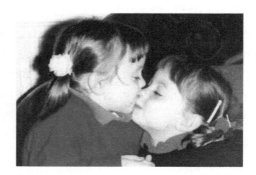
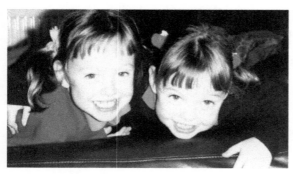

As you can see: fun and giggling were my girl's priority!

Chapter 12) My personal story - How I planned to have twins

This is my personal story. This chapter is about how I achieved my dream: giving birth to identical twin daughters.

I was 33 when I started to try to get pregnant and my husband was 44. My height was 1m65 / 5.4 ft my weight was 65kg / approx. 10 stone so I wasn't fat or obese.

My husband already had 4 children from his previous marriage when I met him.My husband had a vasectomy reversal 3 months prior to when we were trying to have twins so we didn't even know if he could produce children. That's the reason why we also practised a few things that can make man's sperm healthier.

My girls were born premature by caesarean at 8 months. My smallest baby was 1,5kg (approx. 3 pounds) and my biggest baby was 2,5kg (approx. 5 pounds). Very often, when twins weigh differently at birth, they catch up when they are older. Funny enough, now at 21, my daughter who was the smallest when born is now just that tiny little bit bigger than her twin sister. So she did indeed catch up!

You have read a lot of different methods in this book about how to increase your chances of getting pregnant and how to increase your chances of having twins. Perhaps some of them will work for you.
In this last chapter, I am explaining what has worked for me.

101

I do not have any twins in the family and I KNOW I had twins because of what I did; I combined the different methods explained in this book. Maybe this combination of methods will not work for you, but I am forever grateful they've worked for me and I want to share them with you. Some of the things that I did are now believed to be against the chances of getting girls, but that is 21 years later and a lot of research has been done since then.

Please realise that none of this is proven to work and some people laugh at it but I know it worked for me.

True, it has to be said, it wasn't "passionate sex" at all times during those days as we had to "do it" as many times as possible. It felt more like a production line but that's indeed what it was: a production line to make something and the end result was the most beautiful thing we have ever made: 2 beautiful, healthy, intelligent identical twin daughters. My dream came true!
I will NEVER forget the day my doctor told me I had twins. I knew I was pregnant but I was really worried as I had a lot of stomach pains/cramps so I went to the doctor. The doctor told me " Oh, the cramps you have is normal for twins". I couldn't believe it! I was going to have twins! It all worked! I started crying - tears of joy.

My husband couldn't believe it either when I told him! I told him over the phone as he was away from home in Toronto on a business trip. He said "book a plane and come over". So I did! I had to share my joy with my husband! That's the reason why I will always associate the Niagara Falls with being sick as when I flew over and we went to see the Niagara Falls, I was literally sick over the water. Nice memories forever.

I got married in December, I started "trying to have twins" in January and my twin girls were born, 1 month premature, in November. So, within 2 months of trying, I was pregnant.

Thank you, to the best husband in the world who kept working on the production line until we had the desired result! A greater love like ours, I believe, does not exist. I love you deeply, with all my heart and soul.

Lots of people say twins are double the trouble. I have never agreed with that. For me, they are double the pleasure and they always will be.

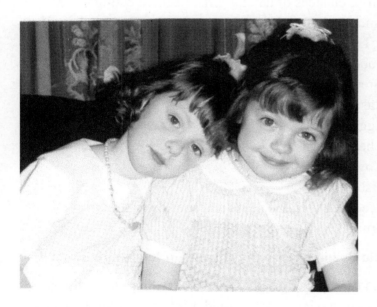

Cute in pink.

I have listed here what I did, starting a few months before we tried to conceive.

You will see that I've already discussed all these methods. When I did my research 22 years ago, I just picked out the methods that I believed in most and that made most sense to me to decide what I was going to practice.

1) Eat food to increase the chances of having girls.

As I wanted twin girls, I used to eat everything that is said to influence your chances of having girls. I started eating these approx. 3 months before I wanted to get pregnant. I used to eat these a lot, I mean 5 times a day or so:

- Food with high levels of magnesium and calcium.
- Green vegetables e.g. broccoli and spinach.
- Raspberries, blueberries, cherries.
- Eggs.
- Cheese.
- Yoghurt.
- Fish.
- Seeds e.g. Sesame seeds and sunflower seeds.
- Fruit.

2) Drink fluids to increase the chances of having girls.

As I wanted twin girls, I used to drink everything that influences your chances of having girls. I would drink these a lot, I mean, a lot, like 5 times a day or so. I started drinking these approx. 3 months before I wanted to get pregnant:

- Milk.
- Runny yoghurts.

3) No tight underwear for the man.

My husband wore loose underwear starting 3 months before we started to try and get pregnant. The reason behind this is that too much heat can lower sperm count. Therefore, if a man wears tight underwear, the temperature of his testicles might be higher and might reduce sperm count. The scrotum is made to hang to keep testicles cooler compared to your body temperature.

4) No hot baths for the man.

My husband "was not allowed" to have hot baths. Sitting in a hot bath can over heat a man's testicles and so kills sperm. So, keep the balls cool.

5) No tight trousers for the man.

My husband "was not allowed" to wear tight jeans because it presses a man's scrotum against his skin. This, again, can overheat the testicles, thus killing sperm.

6) No alcohol for either woman or man.

Neither husband nor me consumed any alcohol from the moment we started trying until the moment I knew I was pregnant. We hardly ever drink alcohol anyway but we were never going to drink any during the months we tried and of course never during the pregnancy.

7) No caffeine for either woman or man.

My husband and me would not drink any caffeine drinks, starting 3 months before we started trying. I gave up coffee and my husband gave up his so much loved coke.

8) Stop taking the contraceptive pill.

I stopped taking the contraceptive pill just before we started trying. Stopping talking it will influence your hormones. A woman is most fertile when she first comes off of the pill.

9) Have a lot of sex in the morning.

We used to have sex a lot in the morning, during fertile days, as sperm concentration might be higher then.

10) Know your ovulation day.

As this is a very important point, I'll repeat here what I've already said in this book. Finding your most fertile days is extremely important.
I took my body temperature every day for a few months to find out when were my most fertile days.

To find out when you ovulate, subtract 14 days from the length of your cycle.

If you have a 28-day cycle, you will ovulate around day 14.
If you have a 25-day cycle, you will ovulate around day 11.
If you have a 35-day cycle, you will ovulate around day 21.

Below is the ovulation chart I used to keep. This document is over 21 years old but I always kept it as I knew, one day, I would write this book.

I was already pregnant in April but didn't know until May. However I stopped taking my temperature at the end of April, as my breasts felt different so I thought I was pregnant.

DATE	JAN	FEBR	MAR	APR
1			36,0	36,2
2				36,3 M
3				36,2 M
4			36,3	35,9 MH
5			36,7	36,5 L
6				35,7 LB
7		35,4		35,9 M
8		36,0		36,0 M
9		36,0		?
10		36,1		36,2 L
11		36,3		35,9 TL
12		36,3		36,7
13		36,3		36,8
14		36,2		36,4
15		36,2	35,9	
16		36,1	36,0	
17		36,4	36,3 36,5	
18		36,3	36,5 ML	34,5 6
19		36,4	?	36,8
20		36,5	36,9 M	36,7
21		35,9	36,7 ML	36,8
22		36,5	36,4 ML	36,5
23		36,5	36,2	36,5
24		36,2	36,4	36,5
25		35,9	36,1 M	36,6
26		35,5	36,4	36,6
27		36,2		36,7
28		36,3	35,8	36,3
29		35,8	35,9 M	36,6
30			36,1	36,7
31			36,2 M	

107

After a woman ovulates, the egg will survive for only approx. 24 hours but sperm can live up to 5 days. This is the reason why you can increase your chances of getting pregnant two to three days before you ovulate. Don't wait to have sex until the day you ovulate, as a man's sperm lives longer than a woman's egg. This means that an egg is often fertilised by sperm that has been in your body a few days before your egg was released. For you to get pregnant, a sperm must fertilise your egg.

Nowadays, some people say that the temperature method is not reliable, however now you can buy ovulation predictor kits.

11) Have sex as many times as humanly possible.

During those most fertile days, we would have sex as many times as humanly possible. My husband would determine the number of times. Sperm production can be compared to producing breast milk: if you use more, you produce more.

12) Have sex in a fertile sex position.

Each time we had sex, it was in one of these three positions:
- Doggy style:

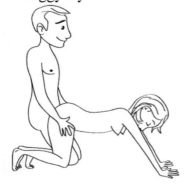

- Rock 'n' Roller:

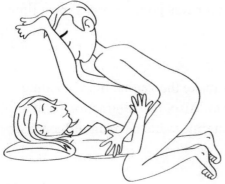

- Missionary:

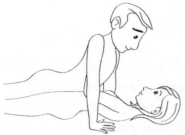

As a result of these positions, there is deep penetration. By getting closer to the cervix during sex, the sperm can swim easier to their target. Lots of people now believe that the missionary position is the best position to conceive girls and the doggy style and Rock 'n' Roller are certainly positions to increase your chances of getting pregnant.

13) Man to stay inside after ejaculation.

After ejaculation, my husband would remain inside me for a few minutes and withdraw slowly and carefully.

14) Woman to stay in the same position for 30 minutes.

After each ejaculation, I would stay in the same position we had sex in. In the case of the doggy position, I was on my hands and knees, head down for at least 30 minutes, usually 45 minutes or even up to one hour. When the hour was gone, it was almost time to start on the next "sex round".

15) No orgasm for the woman!

It is known that female orgasms make the vagina more alkaline and that is not good for girl sperm. Also, the contractions that are produced during orgasm in the uterine walls have an influence on boys or girls sperm.

16) Take Folic Acid

Three months before we decided to start trying for a baby, I started to take a Folic Acid supplement.

17) Believe it can happen.

"Whatever the mind can conceive and believe, it can achieve" is a famous quote by Napoleon Hill. I practice this in business and in everyday life but I also practiced it in achieving twins. I always said to myself: " I WILL have identical twin girls". I never said to my friends: "We are trying for a baby", instead, I always said: "We are trying for twins and we will have them".

Whether my belief has played a role or not I will never know but I do know I believed it and I achieved it!

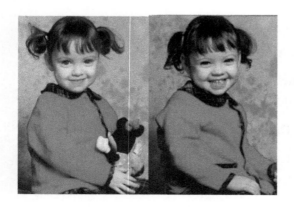

Chapter 13) The pleasures of being a twin

This chapter of the book is written by Amelia and Sandra, my twin daughters.

It really is a pleasure to be born a twin, and much more so to have an identical twin sister who is also your best friend. The twin bond is more enduring than any other relationship on earth, starting even before birth, and often outlasting many friendships and even marriages.

A twin is someone with whom you can share every stage of your life. Whatever you are going through, be it bodily or hormone changes, boyfriend/girlfriend and friend troubles, exams or jobs, there is always someone in the exact same situation as you are. The natural stages that one goes through in life are shared and fully understood by the closest person to you and the things you worry or stress about will be the exact same things that your twin worries and stresses about. Therefore, you always have someone to talk to about these problems. Sharing the stressful stages together offers a comfort.

Sharing milestones is a joy. Sharing the same stressors is one thing, but sharing the most memorable and character building moments in your life with your twin is and has been a wonderful experience for the two of us. Working towards goals can often cause a competitive nature, but in our experience this has always been healthy, and has only encouraged our success. Milestones such as being accepted into grammar school, as well as university and internships, passing exams and driving tests, were all amazing moments in themselves, but knowing that someone shares your joy at the same time, and being happy for each other is a whole different experience.

111

It is much more than being physically there to talk to; twins, we feel, have a special bond that no one else can understand. It is true that living in the same house makes it convenient to talk to your twin and they are unavoidable, but for us this bond is deeper. From experience, it can upset the people closest to you to think that you have an even deeper connection, which no one can come between or understand, with someone else. Of course, some twins do not get on, but from our experience it is a pleasure to have someone to talk to and who understands you better than yourself. Similarly, if we feel that we need to get something off our chests, we can always trust each other not to tell anybody else. How can you explain how we could never stay annoyed at each other and made up really quickly without saying anything? It is that unique bond and understanding that we share that makes this possible. Or maybe it is because we wanted to borrow some shoes the next day.

Another good thing about being a twin is that we have never been bored at home. As previously stated, there is always someone there of your age to do things with. For example, a lot of people told us that they used to wish that their best friend from school lived with them, that way the fun would never end. Those who were an only child would feel this jealousy more strongly, and we could never imagine not having someone there constantly. We never experienced this because our best friend was always there, in the same house, to have fun with or to do nothing with. Not to forget there was always an extra wardrobe there…

Sharing our own private jokes and our own language would brighten up any moment. Of course these things can be shared with friends and siblings, but being a twin, you can create whole different dimensions. While the twin bond is special and unique, it is often endowed with supernatural qualities, and pretending to have twin telepathy and discovering 'evidence' to make people believe this was always our favourite. We also used to love using our own special language to talk about people when they were right there or to tell the other something that we didn't want everyone to hear. Figuring out tricks to always say the same number as each other when asked which one we were thinking of always freaked people out, but to us it was hilarious. It somehow strengthened our unique twin bond. We remember when one twin had an operation on their ear, the other twin was going around school 'in pain', as her 'ear was hurting as she felt every step of the operation'. We will never stop laughing about the reactions we evoked with that joke! You can even start private jokes before birth, as I (Amelia) am often reminded that I was the one who stole her food in the womb, and for that, I owe my sister for life.

Having a twin also makes it easier to be empathetic. A lot of twins are more than just genetically identical; they have the same personalities and interests too. We, personally, have not experienced this, but it is in no way a bad thing. We each have very different interests; one is into neuroscience, the other, languages, for example. Having different personalities is actually a good thing, as it helps you to learn to understand how different people act or react to certain situations. Spending so much time with someone who is very different to you, and still getting along with them, teaches us how to feel empathy for another person's situation or feelings, even if we do not feel the same. We have learnt this from an early age and it has gone on to help us in later life.

Being a twin makes you feel different, more interesting and special compared to others. It is true; a lot of attention comes with being a twin. In our younger years, wearing the same outfit, having the same hairstyle, and especially the same shoes, was always something we took pride in (mainly because it stopped people from telling us apart). We loved to create mirror images of each other, and we always walked side by side, everywhere we went. We wanted everyone to know that we were one. We were 'the twins'. As we grew older, the wrong name calling became more of a nuisance, and we diversified in every way imaginable, from appearance to interests. As we met new people and started new lives, it was bizarre to interact with people who didn't know you as a twin, but your own person, but we still knew that we would always be one. It is a strange compatibility that no one can break, no matter how different you are.

As with any other relationship, twins can argue, disagree and bicker (mainly because we've never had our own birthday)! But the making up part never took long, as being distant from each other felt like something was missing. We have never known loneliness, and for as long as we both live, we never will.

Thank you Mum, for not only doing everything you could to have us but also for doing everything humanly possible to make us happy and to give us good lives. We know you work a lot and that you feel guilty for that, but we understand that everything you do is for us. Thank you Dad, for the hospital trips when we were younger and for always being there to talk to (or if we are ever in need of a sarcastic comment!) We know that we can always come to you, whatever problem we have.

You have both taught us everything we know about how to be a good person, about work ethic, the value of money and most importantly about the value of family. The most important thing that you have taught us is « never let anything come between family, whatever the problem is, you can solve it » and we truly abide by this worldly advice.

To the best parents ever, we love you,

Amelia and Sandra

Chapter 14) The pleasures of being a twin parent

1) From a mum to her daughters.

How do you start to tell the people who made your dream come true how thankful you are? I have no idea! In this chapter I wish to thank my two daughters, Amelia and Sandra and I wish to tell them how much they mean to me.

Normally, I would write something for each one of my daughters, but as this is a book, I am writing something that applies to both of them. The guilty feeling as a parent of twins kicks in again here: I don't want to write something different to both my girls, just in case, one sounds more "loving" than the other.

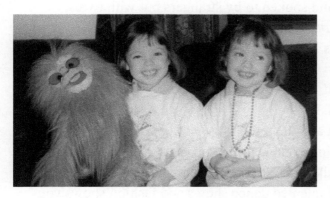

It is hard to find a picture when they were not smiling!

To my daughters:

You truly are the most amazing daughters any mum could wish for. I can't believe it was 21 years ago that my dream came true and you were both born.

A greater love from a mum towards her children, I believe, does not exist. I love you deeply, with all my heart and soul. I know it is your dream to have identical twin daughters- better start the production line as soon as you are ready!

What have been my greatest pleasures? Gosh, where do I start? I'll sum up a few pleasurable things that will stay in my memories forever.

- Wherever I was, people would stop, stare and ask questions like "Are they twins?" or "What beautiful twins you have!" or "How are you coping with twins?". It is a fact, people with single babies are not stopped and spoken to by strangers but with twins, strangers just start talking.
- The tremendous fun I had seeing you play with each other for hours and hours.
- Your first steps!
- Your first words!
- Your first tooth and the tooth fairy giving you money for it!
- The incredible joy I had hearing you giggling and laughing with each other and talking in your own language.
- The amazingly talented dance shows and fashion shows you have performed.
- Your "hyperactive" hour each and every time you had a McDonalds meal.
- The pleasure I have in seeing that you both love each other and want to see each other as much as you can, even now that your lives have their own paths.

- Your performances at the summer dance school.
- The lovely cards you drew for us.
- Your piano playing at the school's music concert.
- Your acting at the school's yearly events.
- The holidays with your niece when I used to dress you as "my triplets" and we used to tell everyone that you were triplets.

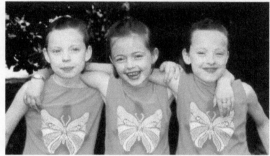

- The frequent stars for excellent achievements you received at school. I can still visualise them on the fridge.
- The fun you had with your birthday parties, with over 30 kids sleeping over!
- Watching Mrs Doubtfire together with dad
- Scaring you with the Child Catcher.
- Your performance as "The Cheeky Girls"

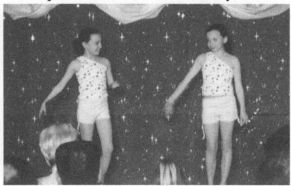

- Your great achievements and positive reports from school.

- You passing your exams for your driving licence.
- Your acceptance in the university of your choice.
- The nerves I had each time you went to a school disco, being worried sick, for nothing.
- Your first boyfriends that I "interviewed" to approve of them.
- Your enormous thrills you used to get, listening to a new audio story at bedtime.
- The stunning views of your looks when you are "dressed up", ready for a party.
- Your excellent results at university.
- The absolute pleasure of bringing you up, giving you values in life and seeing that you have absorbed all the things I thought you.

I look forward to you being married and having twins, if you still want twins. Who knows!

I am pasting below a copy of the poem I wrote to both of you, when you were leaving home to live on your own for your studies. I think the poem sums it all up nicely.

To my dearest darling daughter,

20 years ago was the best day of my life; you arrived on this earth,
and I even fulfilled my dream with a multiple birth.
I've tried to teach you what's right and wrong,
I've also told you that you always have to be strong,
because life will throw things at you that are not nice,
and unfortunately you can't just throw the dice
to make difficult decisions that matter
and nobody will give you the solution on a silver platter.

118

I've tried to warn you about the dangers surrounding you wherever you are,

as you already know, some people are simply just horrible and bizarre.

I've tried to tell you to believe what you see, not what you hear, guess you're now old enough to know that, my dear, go forward with no fear.

I've tried to make you realise you that you can't always believe what people say,

just check it out in your own intellectual way.

I've tried to inform you that sometimes you have to accept things out of your control,

In that case, move on and just keep fighting for your goal.

I've tried to show you to make the best out of a bad situation, just decide things based on your higher education.

I've tried to make you see that happiness and health are more important than money,

although often you need money to be happy, honey.

I've tried to tell you not to trust anyone,

but keep to your track and do what must be done.

I've advised you to eat a mixture of the 5 groups of food, it will do your mind and body good.

I can only hope all my lessons and advice will travel with you, wherever you are and whatever you will do.

Never forget I will always support you whatever decisions you make,

even if it turns out to be a mistake.

If you ever need any help or advice,

come to me, don't even think twice.

Although you will be miles away,

you can contact me any time of the day.

I am so proud of you for who you are and what you have become so far,

you are my star.
May you meet love, happiness, health and lastly money,
I will miss you my honey!
All in all, I've tried to give you a flying start,
because I love you with all my heart.
Whatever life brings,
always see the bright side of things.
Good luck my dear daughter,
Your biggest supporter, EVER

2) From a dad to his daughters.

This small section is written by my husband, proud father of our identical twin daughters. He has always been a man of few words.

"Ever since the day I was told that we were expecting twins it has created a special bond between my wife and the two girls that came into my life.

It has never been a problem to look after two and in my mind no extra work or hassle, just a most fulfilling and wonderful time getting to know and bringing up two exceptional ladies!
I feel a very strong bond to my twin daughters who have greatly enhanced my life.

Anyone that is privileged enough to be the father of twins is a very lucky person."

Chapter 15) Practical advice from a twin parent

1) Generally speaking

Although everyone is different, and everything you've read in this book will help you be extremely prepared, there are still a few more tips I'd like to share.

I've probably mentioned them a bit previously, but I want to emphasize them now.

- Take time for your partner. Having two children at the same time can wipe you out if you're not careful. You don't want to change the dynamics so severely that you lose the essence of your relationship, right? It really is important to find ways to have time to spend alone, just the two of you.

- Getting help - it might sound impossible, but it is hugely important. You may have to trade babysitting time with another couple. You may have to exchange favours with a trusted friend. If you can afford it, using a nanny or trusted babysitter would work well on a regular basis.

- Night nurse - Again, if you have the budget get the help of a night nurse. You will keep your sanity, your health and your humour without stress. Of course, there are disadvantages, but is an excellent expense if you feel it's affordable. No need to be said, that you have to do all the work if you breast feed. Every 3 hours you will have to feed 2 babies.

- Spend time with each baby - that goes for both you and your partner. You'll want to get to know each one individually right from the beginning.

- Join groups - others who have multiple births will be going through the same things. Sharing resources, ideas and anecdotes will help all of you.

- Unsolicited advice - never a good thing under any circumstances, particularly now. Find a way to gently tell your advisor that you appreciate it, but are handling things differently.

- Expect to see life as you've never known it - the first 6 months will make you feel like there will never be a light at the end of the tunnel. But it does get easier!

- Join a playgroup - you will need to get out of the house and so will the babies. Getting involved in a local playgroup will expand your world and make you a better-rounded mother and person.

- Online answers - more than ever before, you can quickly find groups, parents and answers on the Internet, when you don't have time.

- Online forums - Twin forums can be comforting and offer ideas and answers you might not find anywhere else. Sometimes the other mothers will give you ideas that save time and money.

- Once your babies are old enough, go to a "Twin Day" that twins from all over the world go to. Search online where they are.

- Continue some sort of exercise, like yoga, and as the kids grow you might even be able to take them to the gym and put them in the day care for an hour. Anything you can do to remain sane and upbeat will help and exercise will be a large part of that.

- If you are first time parents, you will make mistakes. Heck, you'll make mistakes even if you have had other children. So go easy on yourselves. Try to realize that no one is perfect.

- Come to some agreements - you and your husband could be outplayed by twins, so be smart and make sure your guidelines and rules are in agreement as the kids grow.

- Enjoy and record every second with your twins. It's a unique experience that will touch you deeply as you watch them interact and grow together. It is extremely satisfying and has made my life what it is today: a happy life full of happy memories.

- You might get a little bit frustrated when they cry and you don't know what to do. Just treasure those moments, as before you know it, they will be adults. Take it all with a smile and then you will have nothing but happy memories to keep with you for the rest of your life. Learn your babies' cries and what they mean, discussed later when I give my own practical advice.

- Your hormones will get messed up. Make sure your husband is aware of it. With a single pregnancy, a woman's hormones are messed up for a while and it might take several months to get back to normal. With a twin pregnancy, your hormones might get messed up even more. Be prepared for it and you will be able to deal with it. In my case, my hormones never really went back to how they were before I got pregnant. Since my girls were born, I struggled with my hormones for about 15 years! Yes, 15 years! I had tablets, patches, oestrogen patches, progesterone patches, a coil, etc. I started my menopause when I was 38. Did it have anything to do with my twin pregnancy? I will never know and no one knows the answer to that but I've got the feeling it did. It was well worth it though as I've got 2 twin daughters for it.

- Persevere with breast milk. In the beginning, it was not easy for me to produce enough milk but I persevered and I was able to feed my babies for 6 months.

Talking about breast milk, it wasn't easy for my husband. Yes, you did read that right: it wasn't easy for my husband. Let me tell you what happened.

One of my girls' lungs was not developed enough when she was born and she was transferred to a specialised lung hospital.

This was the situation the first 10 days after my girls were born:

- I was in hospital

- One girl in one hospital-the same hospital I was in

 - The other girl in another hospital

I would breast feed my baby that was with me in the hospital and I would use a breast pump to make milk in a bottle for my other baby. That milk was transported by my husband, every 3 hours to the baby that was in the lung hospital. So, every 2 hours, my husband would start his 30-minute journey there, drop off the milk, quickly admire his daughter, and come back home for another 30-minute journey back to the hospital. He rested for about 30 minutes and started his way back to the hospital with another bottle of milk. He never wanted to risk getting stuck in a traffic jam, so he always left extra early.

This was the situation 10 days after the birth:

I was allowed to go home. So:

- I was home

- One daughter was still in the hospital where she was born, as she was still in the incubator, being premature and under weight. I'll call this hospital: Hospital 1.

- The other daughter was still in the lung hospital. Hospital 2.

I would stay at home, pumping milk all the time into 2 bottles this time. My husband would leave on his 30-minute journey to hospital 1 to drop off one bottle of milk, quickly admire his daughter, leave the hospital and continue his journey to hospital 2, which was another 15 minutes drive. Quickly drop off the bottle with milk and quickly admire his other daughter, and then on his way back home, a 45-minute drive. He would rest at home for maximum 1 hour and then leave again with another 2 bottles of milk to start his journey to hospital 1 and hospital 2 again. In the beginning, my girls needed fresh breast milk every 3 hours. There simply was not enough time for my husband to give the milk (from the bottle) so the nurse used to do it. The most important thing for my husband and me was that they got the breast milk, however it was given to them.

Can you believe my husband did this for 3 full months: driving milk up and down! Three full months, day AND night! I do admire him.

This was the situation 1 month after the birth:

The daughter that was not in the lung hospital was allowed to come home after one month of being born as she did put on enough weight to come home.

So:

- I was home

- One of my daughters was home

- One of my daughters was still in the lung hospital.

So it got a little bit easer for my husband and for me. I could give breast milk at home to one baby, pump the rest into a bottle and my husband only had to drive to one hospital again.

3 months after birth, my babies were both home so I could breast-feed them both at home.

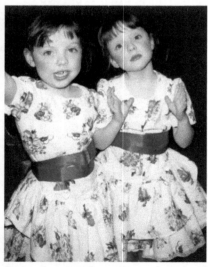

Just practiced putting some make up on!

2) My own personal ways have worked

Now that I have mentioned some general tips in this chapter, I am going to share some basic education principles that I believe in and that I have practiced bringing up my twin daughters.

Some people call twins "Double Trouble". I have always hated that quote. I always use to say to people that they are "Double The Fun" and each time I said it, I meant it.

Every child needs discipline, rules, routines and consistency but for twins, you will definitely have to apply these. These "education rules" also apply if you only have one baby.
I am not a sergeant, which you might think when you read my advice on the following few pages. Instead, I do believe you have to be hard to be kind in some situations when bringing up children, because that way they know they are surrounded by people who love them and in the end want only the best for them.

I am in no way a child education expert but I see myself as a well-educated woman. During my pregnancy I read tons of books about the education of children and of twins and I have put the principles that I believed in into practice. The result of that is that I now have 2 respectful young adults as my daughters.

I will not write pages and pages on each topic, as that would fill a whole book. I will just share with you the basic principles that I advise you to do as it worked for me, so it might work for you. Here we go.

a) **Don't wait too long for more children.**

Ideally, I would have liked to have more than 2 children. I made one mistake: waiting too long to have more children. Out of love for my girls, I waited to have more children. Let me explain. At home, everything is usually perfectly OK and manageable with twins. The trouble is going out. You need to take everything in your "just in case" bag: nappies, toys, food, milk, crayons, colouring books, medication perhaps, etc. Now some mums struggle to carry one bag around but you need to carry everything around for 2 children. Imagine this scenario: you are taking your children to a park to play in the playground. There is a little muddy path and it is impossible to push the buggy on that path in order to get to the playground. The only solution is taking the children out of the buggy. OK, that's easy but here comes the tricky bit: pushing the buggy over the muddy path AND holding hands with each one of your children. It simply is not possible! On top of that you have to carry the " just in case" bag full of stuff as when you leave it hanging on the buggy, the buggy will fall over.

I had occasions like this all the time, almost everywhere I went: where it was practically impossible for my children to be SAFE because if I would let go of their hands whilst pushing the buggy forwards with my stomach, in my opinion that meant that my girls were not safe. They were still too young to let go as you never know 1) who snatches them from you and 2) where they all of a sudden run to e.g. a dog in the park that is not friendly with children.

So, for the love I had for my children and my concern for their safety, I decided not to have other children until my twin daughters were 5, when it was easier to look after them in a safe way on my own e.g. they could hold each others hands whilst I would hold one hand and push the buggy, coming back to the playground scenario. Or they could both help me pushing the buggy whilst I would hold their hands.

Unfortunately when they were 5, as I mentioned before, my hormones were still up the creek. I tried to get pregnant again, yes, I was trying for twins again! But it was not meant to be: I had 5 miscarriages and I decided that was a sign for me better not to have more children.

My advice to you: if you want more children, don't delay it as long as I did, as you never know, you might also hit the menopause early. This is unlikely to apply to you if you are only 21 when you are trying to conceive.

b) On demand feeding or not?

On demand feeding means that you feed your babies when they "ask for it" by crying. I personally don't believe in feeding on demand, certainly not for twins. You might be feeding all day. From the moment your babies are born, you need to get a system going. That also means a system for feeding.

So, the opposite of on demand feeding is working with a feeding schedule. When your babies are only just born, that will be every 3 hours.

The downside, only at the very beginning, is that when the time comes to feed, you might have to wake up your babies to feed them. Some people say you shouldn't wake up sleeping babies. I disagree with that. The baby's body will very soon adapt to their feeding schedule and every 3 hours, after a while, they will wake up for their food.

c) Leave them crying

At the beginning, I think it is crucially important to leave your babies crying, for say minimum 20 minutes. They won't know you yet and you don't know them yet. All babies will naturally "test" you to see what happens when they cry, how long they have to cry for to get your attention. It is nicer for them to be in your arms all the time so that's what they will want to achieve, very often, by crying. You know better, you know it is not possible to keep them in your arms all the time therefore you need to tell them that they can't have what they want, when they want it and you need to establish the rules, starting immediately.

Here's a scenario from mum A:
- 7PM baby is just put to bed.
- 7.05 PM baby cries and mum goes to pick her up for 10 minutes, holding her and sing songs are cuddle her baby.
- 7.15PM mum puts baby back to bed.
- 7.16PM baby cries, as of course, the baby wants to be cuddled again.
- 7.20PM mum picks baby up again and cuddles baby.
- 7.30 PM mum puts baby back to bed.
- 7.31 PM baby cries again.
- You see where this is going. Mum and the baby can be awake until the early hours in the morning.

Here's a scenario from mum B:
- 7PM baby is just put to bed.
- 7.05 PM baby cries and mum does nothing.
- 7.25PM mum checks, very quietly, entering baby's room to make sure baby is not hot or does not appear to be ill. Mum does not pick up baby and does not say anything and leaves the room.
- 7.26 PM baby cries again. Mum knows nothing is wrong with the baby and lets her cry.
- 7.30PM baby sleeps.

The next day the baby will very likely fall asleep at 7.20PM, the day after at 7.15Pm, etc.

Mum B creates a future with rules and discipline whilst mum A creates a future with crying and possibly later tantrums. Every single night will be a battle between mum A and baby.

Important to mention: scenario B can only be done if you know very well nothing is wrong with the baby:
- No signs of being ill e.g. runny nose, chesty cough.
- No fever.
- No signs of the baby having stomach pains: babies will very often kicks their legs in the air with stomach pain.
- Baby is not too hot.

d) Learn to recognize their cries

It is crucially important that you learn your baby's cries. A baby will cry differently when tired, when hungry, when ill, etc. Make sure you pay attention to the type of cry and analyse everything when they cry. You will soon be able to tell: "that's a hunger cry" or " that's a stomach pain cry", etc. Your 2 babies will likely to have different cries, so you will have to recognise a minimum of six cries!

e) Don't worry about your weight gain.

I personally put on 40 kg (over 6 stone) during my pregnancy and 21 years later I still didn't lose it all! I never went back to the slim figure I had before I was pregnant.

Don't make it a priority to start with to lose the weight quickly, definitely not if you are breast-feeding. You need to eat very healthily as you have 2 babies to feed.

Worry about losing weight when you've stopped breast-feeding.

f) Your stomach

If you are like me, you might still have a "twin" stomach after 21 years. I never got rid of my stomach. I mean, it doesn't look disgustingly fat but I know I will always have a "twin" stomach but I don't mind. I've got it because of my girls and they are well worth it. Now, I must admit that I have never seriously tried to get rid of my stomach because I always had more important things to do. The fact that I have the best husband in the world, who actually loves me for who I am, probably has something to do with it.

Don't get depressed about your stomach. Try and lose it if it bothers you. If you can't lose it, just accept it! C'est la vie!

Although I have a stomach, I don't have any stretch marks at all, guess you can never have it all hey!

g) Sleep when they want to sleep

Well, I am a structured person in everything that I do. I knew I would have to get a sleep system going in order for us, my husband and me, to get some sleep.

From the very start, I set up a system e.g. what time they would go to bed, what time I would get them up, etc.... everything was structured. I had diaries for everything: sleeping, playing, eating, bathing, etc. I think this is really important. Everyone gets used to the system, including your babies.

h) Evening routine

You must, must, must set up an evening routine from day 1. These routines will need adjusting, as they grow older, of course. It is of crucial importance that you set up an evening routine. My routine was 1 hour and was as follows:

- 6pm: Bath time. Bath time is fun time, or at least, it was in our house.
- 6.15 pm: pyjamas on and playtime for 15 minutes. We had playtime in our lounge and usually fun times.
- 6.30 pm: Time to read a story in their bedroom, not in the lounge or kitchen. Read a story with a very small light on.
- 6.45 Time to kiss them goodnight and tell them I love them.
- After I left the room, they were allowed to listen to another story that I would play, in those days on a cassette player. Nowadays, you would put a CD on or an MP3 Player.
- 7pm. I would go in and say firmly "time for bed" and switch the music or electronic story off and the lights out.

It's as simple as that. My girls got used to that routine and they loved it.

In the first week or so, you might have to be very firm and tell them off if they are not quiet after "lights out". Just leave them crying for a while and they will soon get the message that when you say "time for bed", you mean it.

Of course, that is why it is so important to learn their cries, as it could be that they are crying because they are ill, in that case, of course, you can go and see them.
If they are crying just because they want to see you, you go back in, don't switch the light on, don't pick them up and simply say firmly: "time for bed".

i) 7PM means 7PM

If your babies usually go to bed at 7PM, put them to bed at 7PM. A lot of parents make the mistake and take their children to a neighbour's party or to the pub, or to late family visits, etc. I have never done that. If we had to go out, to a pub or a party, I would make sure I had a baby sitter so my girls could stay in their evening routine.

A lot of parents put themselves first or put their own pleasures before their duty of being a responsible parent. They will go to a party because it is a "Not to be missed party" and they take their children with them, taking them out of their usual routine. I totally agree with that, your children should come first and if you can't get a babysitter, you simply don't go to the party.

Never would my babies be seen after 7PM before the age of 3, other than at home. Of course, the odd exceptions were allowed e.g. when travelling.

j) You must have a routine

Children need routines, children love routines and children mostly behave extremely well with routines.
- Make a routine for the morning.

- Make a scheduled time for lunchtime.
- Make a routine for the afternoon.
- Make a scheduled time for evening meal.
- Make a routine for the evening.

I don't think I have ever interrupted my routines for anything. I would arrange my whole life around my routines, as I knew it would make my girls happy and it would make life easy for everyone involved.

k) I don't like it!

Here's another mistake I think a lot of parents make who have more than one child.

You have prepared a meal and are about to give it to your twins. One of them loves it and one of them says "I don't like it". So you say: "OK darling, I will make you something else". By doing this, you will create a problem at food times for the rest of your life or at least, for as long as you are feeding your children.

Here's what I said when one of my girls said "I don't like it". I reply: "Ok, no problem don't eat it then but the next time you will get food will be in 4 hours time so if you're hungry, that's tough. You know you won't get a snack if you don't eat your main meals".

Maybe, just maybe your child might be a little bit hungry until the next mealtime. That won't harm the child at all. You've got to be hard to be kind. You've got to be hard once, maximum 3 times, to be kind. Putting down the rules firmly pays off for everyone.

l) Snack routines

Yes, even for snacks, biscuits, crisps, I had routines. This was a typical day in our house:

AM

- 7 rise and shine and have a giggle or a play

- 7.15 breakfast

- 7.45 get dressed

- Playtime

- 10 time for a snack e.g. grapes, apple, raisins, etc. When the girls were older, it would now and again be a biscuit or some crisps. You can't keep the sweets away forever!

- 12 lunch

PM

- 12.30 playtime

- 2 snack time

- 5 dinner

- 6 time to start evening routine

-7 lights out and time for bed

Of course, these routines can change but young children adapt to any situation quickly.

My girls would always know what to expect and when to expect it.

You will see if you practice it yourself: routines will make your children happy and they will make the parents happy.

m) 10 minutes rule

Imagine you are preparing a meal. Your husband comes in and says: "Come on, we are leaving right now". You wouldn't be happy, you would say: "Hang on, let me just finish peeling the carrots". He replies: "now please". You definitely wouldn't be happy!

Children are always doing something as well! They are thinking or playing or reading but in their own little world they are doing something. They don't like to be interrupted in whatever they are doing but lots of mums do it. They say: "Put your coat on, we are going now". The child cries, to tell you, in a way "I am doing this now, just wait a minute". The mum replies: "I said, now, put your coat on".

The child thinks you are horrible and you think your child doesn't listen to you.

Situations like that are not pleasant for child or parent but there is a very easy solution: the 10-minute rule.

Always tell your children in advance what you are planning to do e.g. "Darling, in about 10 minutes we need to go and see Auntie Emily so can you finish what you are doing so you are ready in 10 minutes". This makes a huge difference in your child's behaviour because your child can, in their own little world think: "Ok, I've got 10 minutes, I'll quickly finish colouring in this part of the drawing and then I can do the rest later".

n) The naughty step works

When your child behaves badly, you can put him/her on the naughty step. In my case, I used to put my children in the corner instead, with their face facing the corner of the walls. Usually it is one minute for every year. So, 2 minutes in the corner for a 2-

year-old, 3 minutes for a 3-year-old, etc.

The child is not allowed to come out of the corner unless the minutes are up. From memory, I've put my children in the corner 5 times in their lifetime. If you are consistent, they will soon avoid having to be put in the corner.

o) Consistency - consistency - so important!

You can make your life so much easier if you are consistent at all times, without exceptions. Children like to live in a predictable environment. It gives them security. When bedtime is one day 7pm and another day 9pm, they become confused. Make sure you pay attention not to become an inconsistent parent. If you make rules, you have to stick to them. If your child asks: "Can I have a biscuit" and you say no, it has to be no. Your child might cry because he/she wants a biscuit. Lots of parents give in and in the end the parent says: "Ok, here is your biscuit". I cannot stress enough how wrong this is. You said no the first time so you have to stick to your no, no matter how much the child cries for their biscuit.

Does your partner say yes to something and you say no? That is also confusing for the child and that way, you will cause friction between you and your partner. You both have to agree in advance what is allowed and what is not.

If you make threats to your children, you have to act upon them. If you say: "If you do that one more time, you are going on the naughty step" then, if the child does it again, you have to put them on the naughty step.

Your children will test your boundaries, so you have to be consistent in everything you do or say.

Consistency makes children feel safe, as they know what to

expect. Your child will be a better student and a better employee or employer when discipline is consistent.

If you are not consistent, your child will test the rules more often and see how far he can go, creating more difficult times for you and for them.

p) Rules and discipline

As you must already know by now, I love rules and regulations, because they are so important. Explain all the rules in your house clearly. Children need limits; they find security in having boundaries.

Make sure you explain the rule in a way that your child understands what is involved. I always used to ask my girls to repeat the rules to me, to make sure they understood. It is also very important that you explain the reason for the rule. I hate the words "Because I told you so" and I have never used them.

Explain the consequences if the rules are not obeyed and it is always a good idea to give your child a choice. Example: "Please pick up your toys". I would ask once more and add "If you don't pick up your toys, I will take them away and won't be able to play with them for 2 days". This clearly gives a choice: pick up the toys or face the consequence and not play with them for 2 days. This is where consistency comes in again: you have to hide the toys for 2 days if the toys are not picked up.

Discipline is very important for a child to feel safe and loved.

If consistency has been applied a few times, most kids will choose to follow the rules. As they grow older, your children will realize that all the rules are set up for their own wellbeing. They see that they can rely on their parents and they know that the parents are looking after them well, by applying rules, discipline and consistency.

q) Let them sort it out.

Very often, children fight over things and twins are no exception. On a regular basis, one of my children would tell me: "Amelia took my toy and I had it first". Now I wasn't there when it happened so I don't really know if Sandra did indeed have the toy first. I think punishing the wrong child is really not a good thing to do at all. So, if I would punish Sandra for having taken the toy, and she didn't do it, that would really not be nice for Sandra.

Instead, I always used to say: "Sort it out amongst yourselves, you started the fight, so you solve it". Of course, I would always watch in the distance how they would sort it out and surprisingly enough, they always used to sort it out amongst them without my help.

This way, they also learn how to solve silly little problems, which is good for them. As you know, they'll have to sort out lots of problems when they're adults!

Never take sides with one child, in case you are wrong. If you didn't see or hear exactly what happened, don't stand in between them and let them sort it out.

r) It's only a phase!

That was my husband's favourite thing to tell me: "It's only a phase" and you know what, he was right all the time.

Sometimes, like every parent, you will have moments where it is all a bit too much. You are not having a good day, your hormones are playing up, you feel ill, etc. On days like that, you get a little bit frustrated if your children are playing up or not listening immediately. As I've already mentioned, they will test your boundaries all the time. On days like this, just think about this:

"It's only a phase"! It will help. I know it did help me.

s) Don't call them twins

You might be surprised by this as I have been talking about twins all the time in this book but I actually never called my girls "the twins" or "my twins". That sounds like they are only one. But, don't forget there are 2 people involved, not one. They have their own personalities, their own desires, their own views on things, so they need to be referred to as 2 different human beings.

The reason why I talk about twins all the time in this book is...well because it is a book about twins.

I always used to call my daughters: my daughters, my girls, Amelia and Sandra. I never used to refer to them to anyone as "the twins". It teaches them from day one that they are 2 different people, which I think is very important for when they become adults.

t) Don't dress them the same when they're older.

I guess this one might surprise you as well as on all the pictures in this book my girls are wearing the same outfit.

That's why it says in the title: "Don't dress them the same when they're older". Of course, dressing them the same when they're young is very cute. People stare at them all the time and you can proudly show off your children. They look absolutely adorable.

However, there comes a time where you have to stop dressing them the same, for their own good. I stopped dressing my children the same when they were about 5 years old.

Why is this important? I guess you can compare it with why I don't call my daughters "The twins". They are 2 children with their own personalities; they will have their own, probably totally different lives. They will have to make their own decisions when they are older. At some point, they will also be separated from each other. If you constantly dress them the same and consider them to be one instead of two it will be more difficult for them to separate when they are older. It will be more painful for them. My girls' big separation happened when they both went to do different universities in different towns. They now have their own lives but do miss each other.

u) Ignore the bad, praise the good.

My dad used to go on and on and on when we misbehaved. 5 months after something happened, he still used to bring it up. I used to absolutely hate that. Instead, what I did with my children, and what I advise you to do is ignore the bad stuff, don't keep bringing it up and praise the good stuff.

The bad stuff can be mentioned and lessons learned but don't keep going on and on about it. Often, children, especially when they are over 10-years-old, learn from their own mistakes, without being punished for them.

Whilst not bringing up the past all the time, you must praise the good stuff. And yes, you can and even must praise the good stuff all the time.

Tell your friends: "Wow, my daughter really made a very pretty picture today" or "I am so impressed with my son, he cleaned up his room all on his own today", etc.

Stick their drawings they come home from school with on the fridge and leave them there for a long time and keep praising your children.

v) Stars work

This next point can be combined with my previous point about praising. Each time your child does something really good or is very nice, etc. give him a star to stick on the Star Chart that is hanging on the fridge.

For each 5 stars your child can get together, they will be rewarded with something e.g. $1 / £1. That way, they can also learn about saving money and the value of money as they can find out what they can buy with their money.

w) Birthday cards

Don't buy a birthday card that says "Happy Birthday Twins". They are 2 people so they deserve a birthday card each, not one, as that means they are one person. As you've just read, they are not "The twins"; they are two people.

One problem I had each year though is "buying the same thing but different". I was really happy when my girls were old enough so I could give them money.

To buy birthday presents that were the same but different was always a challenge. When my girls were still young, they were more or less interested in the same toys, the same clothes, etc. Ideally I would want to buy a "Game Boy" for one but another game with the same sort of value for the other. Problem is they both would have wanted the same Game Boy because that was the "in" thing.

Same with clothes: buy one outfit in purple and the same outfit in cream is not always easy as a lot of shops don't sell the same clothes but in a different colour and if you go to a shop for twins, they will sell only the same clothes.

Somehow I managed to make them happy on their birthdays. I never used to over indulge anyway as I did try to teach my girls the value of money.

Then there is the guilt! Yes, the guilt you have when you spend a few pounds more on one child compared to the other. I always used to hate that: when you do try and buy different things, you have to make sure they are the same value otherwise you can't get it over your heart if you give one more than the other. My girls never seemed to think it was a problem, but I did.

x) Get new stuff for trips

One of my last tips is a good one I think. Travelling with children is not easy; long car journeys, train journeys, flights, even going shopping for a few hours are not children's favourite things to do. I always used to take new toys, new colouring books, new games with me each time I would travel somewhere with my girls. That way, when they've had enough and you can feel they are getting a little bit difficult, you present them with something brand new that they will be interested in it.

Lots of parents say: "Just play with your toys" but if all the toys are 2 years old, they won't be very interesting for them. That's why you need to take new stuff on each journey. You might not need it but if you do, you'll be glad you took it.

y) Take each child separately

Now and again, when you can and the opportunity arises, take only one of the twins out, with the other twin left at home.

That way, you achieve 3 things:

- You can pay full attention to one child, as usually there are 2. This will be good for your relationship with the child and you get the chance to bond with only one.

- The child can be on her own, without the other twin being there all the time. This is nice for the child.

- You can take one child out and your husband gets the chance, at home with the other twin, to bond with only one child. The other

144

twin also gets time, just for herself, without the other twin.

z) Tell them you love them

Unfortunately I didn't come from a happy family. My mum or dad never told me they loved me and I did crave that. I was constantly craving love and attention when I was young. Please don't do this to your children. Because I never had it, I made it a point to make sure I told my children every day, before bedtime, that I loved them. It was always the last thing I said, each day: "Love you" and then I heard the reply twice: " Love you". Every single day that made me happy! I am pretty sure it made them happy as well as they knew they were in a loving home.

That's 26 "rules" I advise you to practice. I surprised myself that there are so many!

The most important rule I believe is to be tough to be kind. Lay down some strict rules from the beginning and everyone is happy: children, mum and dad.

The second, most important rule is consistency so everyone knows you mean business if the rules are not followed. I now know that my girls think it was a good way of education. Proof was that my girls were always happy and giggling so they were happy in the "strict" environment that I created for them.

The only thing I have always wanted is for my daughters to be happy and become responsible adults with good values for the future.

Top Tip 1: Don't give twins names starting with the same letter e.g. Tim and Tom or Marion and Mandy. That way, when you have to mark their belongings at home or at school, you can just put the first letter on each item. In my case, on one item I would simply write the letter "A" and an "S" on the other item.

Top Tip 2: Don't have the TV on whilst eating. Having breakfast, lunch or dinner in our house was always fun with my girls. We talked for hours. Lots of families eat dinner from a tray whilst watching TV. I have always been against that. Children these days are concentrating on their electronic devices all the time so they don't talk a lot. No TV, games or phones are allowed in our house whilst we eat. Eating-time is ideal to talk about problems and finding solutions or simply talking about all sorts of things. Telling jokes was also often on our agenda whilst eating.

Chapter 16) Famous twins

We rarely think of celebrities as twins. However, there are quite a few, as you can see from this list.

a) Scarlett and Hunter Johansson

Hunter's acted in a movie with Scarlet and has also been a campaign advisor for President Obama.

b) Ashton and Michael Kutcher

Ashton's brother, Michael, still lives in their home state of Iowa. As a child, Michael was diagnosed with cerebral palsy and had a heart transplant.

c) Aaron and Angel Carter

Brother of Backstreet Boy hunk, Aaron and Angel are fraternal twins, with a strong self-proclaimed twin-ship.

d) Vin Diesel and Paul Vincent

Vin's fraternal brother, Paul, is also in the business. Paul works as a respected film editor and we all know what Vin is capable of.

e) Kiefer and Rachel Sutherland

Kiefer's little seven-minute-later-born sister is also a Hollywood star, although she works in post-production as a supervisor.

f) Gisele and Patricia Bundchen

The famous Brazilian model's twin sister is just as gorgeous.

g) Alanis and Wade Morissette

Twins Wade and Alanis are both singers. Wade is also a yoga instructor and author. Both have sons with same middle name.

h) Tiki and Ronde Barber

Tiki is an on-air personality while Ronde is a football player with the Tampa Bay Buccaneers.

i) Romulus and Remus

Romulus went on to kill his twin brother, Remus, in ancient Rome. This might even be how Rome got its name.

j) Elvis and Jesse Presley

Yes, it's true. Elvis had a birth twin they named Jesse. Jesse was stillborn, while Elvis survived and flourished.

k) Ann Landers and Abigail Van Buren

Twin sisters with twin occupations, these advice columnists spent their lifetime telling others how to run their lives successfully. The odd thing is they were not known to get along very well with one another.

l) Mary Kate and Ashley Olsen

The cute twins from the 80's sitcom Full House have grown up, but will still be remembered for the work they did together.

m) Justin and Laura Timberlake

Justin had a twin sister, Laura, who died at birth.

n) Robin and Maurice Gibb

The well-known group, The Bee Gees, were actually three brothers, but two of them were twins. They sure showed that twins had plenty of harmony.

o) Jacob and Esau

These biblical twins probably own the honour of being the first pair born at the same time. They might not be so well known in modern times, but they sure appeared in a lot of books.

p) Jenna and Barbara Bush

These two might not have done as much to make themselves famous, but being "first twins" was no easy task. They are the fraternal twin daughters of George W. Bush and Laura Bush.

q) The Kray Brothers

Famous London gangsters, these twins were two men you wouldn't want to cross. Ronnie and Reginald were notorious for their violence on one hand and ability to rub elbows with Judy Garland and Frank Sinatra on the other.

r) Chang and Eng Bunker

If you don't recognize the names, you are not alone. The "Siamese Twins" from Siam, Thailand brought attention to the lives of conjoined twins.

s) Parker and Christopher Posey

Actress Parker Posey has a brother who stays far away from the Hollywood scene. Christopher and Parker were brought up in Louisiana.

t) Isabella Rossellini and Isotta Ingrid

Daughters of famous icon Ingrid Bergman, Isabella and Isotta chose two different careers. Isabella went into Italian literature and teaches at Harvard.

u) Jerry Hall and sister Terry

The sisters are and have always been close. Luckily not everything is shared.

v) Joseph and Jacob Fiennes

The actor Joseph Fiennes has a twin who is a game-keeper and conservationist in Norfolk, Virginia. Jacob is a self-proclaimed country boy who likes a more quiet life.

w) Dylan and Cole Sprouse

These twins starred in "Big Daddy" before they had their own TV show.

x) Olly and Ben Murs.

The British singer Olly has a twin brother who was pretty angry when Olly missed his wedding whilst competing on The X-Factor TV show.

y) The Cheeky Girls!

This pop duo released their single in 2002 with "The Cheeky Song (Touch My Bum)". My girls used to love The Cheeky Girls.

There are many more famous twins, just search online. Wikipedia has a large list:
http://en.wikipedia.org/wiki/List_of_twins

Who knows, perhaps my daughters will be listed as "famous twins" in the future! As long as they are happy though, famous or not!

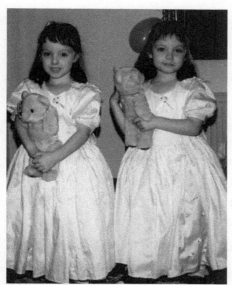

The end of a tiring day at a party.

Chapter 17) Amazing twin stories

A variety of true stories

Identical twins are always the source of curiosity.
The stories we hear depict twins as people who have things
happen simultaneously without any logical reason.
They are also known to be able to feel what the other is feeling,
even when there is a great distance between them.

I don't think the twins are as enamoured with the coincidences
that happen as much as we are. You'll enjoy these stories, as I
handpicked them from the volumes of available tales from around
the world.

a) Even when twins don't share the same colours,
personalities, food choices or hobbies, there seems to be a
connection that keeps them in tune with one another.

b) Recently, when two twins living on different continents
touched base on Skype, they discovered that they both had
purchased the same pair of trousers, in the same colour, at
the same shop. To top that off, they even made the
purchase on the same day!

c) There are more stories of twins buying each other the
exact same CD, calling their mother within five minutes of
one another and buying gifts for others that inadvertently
match. You will enjoy these types of experiences, I'm
sure, as your twins grow.

d) Two boys were given up for adoption at birth, and when
they met for the first time almost 40 years later, they

learned they were both named the same first name as one another: Jim. The adoptive parents never met or spoke.

e) In Finland, two older gentlemen both died in car accidents on the same day. The oddity of the story is that the accidents happened on the same road, a couple of hours apart.

f) In 2004, a young woman gave birth. She had a relationship with one twin, so he thought he was the father. The truth was that she slept with both of the identical twins on the same day. Since they have matching DNA, there is no way to tell which one is really the father.

g) Did you hear the one about the twin sisters who gave birth on the very same day and within two hours of one another? Their due dates were within a week of one another.

h) In a British school in Lincolnshire, there are 20 sets of twins. But the funniest part is the school requires uniforms and most of the twins are in the seventh grade.

i) After 35 years of being separated at birth and adopted by different parents, both girls realized that they had always lived similar lives. Both were school newspaper editors, film students and both became writers.

j) Here's a cute one: When two Chinese girls were selected for adoption from the same agency, the two couples shared photos of the girls with one another. They had met only through common community adoption clubs, and when sharing the photos, they noticed the similarities between the two. The adoption agency assured the women that it was not true, however the women had the DNA tested and learned they were identical twins. Luckily, the families grew close and elected to sort of raise the children together.

k) Injured on the same day - When one twin fell over a slide and went to hospital, he was sent home and told it was nothing. The same day, his twin tripped over the same slide, fell and broke his arm. Both brothers went to the hospital and as it turned out, the first brother also had a broken arm.

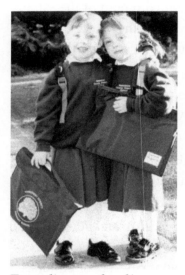

First day at school!

Chapter 18) Twin studies & myths

1) Twin Studies

Most of the studies that have been done about twins have been about whether it is the environment in which they live that determines their similar behaviours or the genetic/biological influences.

We hope in the future that more studies will focus on how to scientifically increase the chances of having twins in the gender of your choice. There is so much to learn about why the twin phenomenon even happens.

The Minnesota Twin Study

This is a well-known study that has four parts: two parts are about identical twins and two are about fraternal twins. The study's primary purpose was to do what we mentioned above - determine whether "twin-ness" is the product of the environment or if it is biological. The way this and similar studies have been done is to use twins who have grown up together and twins who have been separated at different stages.

What they have concluded is that twins who grew up apart are as likely to be similar to their twin counterpart as if they grew up under the same roof.

This clearly states that twins are biologically similar and although environment may play a role in having parallel interests - it is very likely due to their genetics.

2) Amusing myths to disregard

We've all been exposed to stories about twins that are passed off as fact. So much so, that most of us grew up believing them. Well, we're going to debunk these myths for you today, so you will know the scientific realities.

Myth: Twins run in families

Fact: Although it is possible for a family to have a genetic predisposition to having twins, it would be more about the woman's genetic predisposition of releasing more than one egg at a time. That only relates to fraternal twins, as you can see, because identical twins are created from one egg and are not hereditary.

Myth: Twins skip a generation

Fact: There is absolutely no evidence to support this. Not sure where this information came from or how it started, but if you have twins there is no data that suggests your daughter will not be able to birth twins. Based on what we said earlier, if the woman is predisposed to releasing more than one egg, she is predisposed to having twins.

If that is a genetically carried aspect that is passed down, then it is more likely that your daughter would have twins, so it wouldn't skip a year.

Myth: Bad morning sickness means twins

Fact: This is a very personal issue and is all over the board. Some women experience the epitome in morning sickness while others experience nothing. There is no truth to the fact that morning sickness has anything to do with multiple births.

Myth: Twins speak their own secret language

Fact: Of course, as with everything, it depends on the twins. But considering they have been together since they were zygotes, it's likely they can communicate in their own way. As for a secret language - it's surely not a universal "twin" language.

Myth: Pregnancies start as twins and change

Fact: Pregnancy scans have shown that many pregnancies have started with two fertilized eggs, with twins on the way. However, after about 12 weeks, one of the twins doesn't make it and is reabsorbed back into the tissue.

There is a name for this: vanishing twin syndrome and as sad as it sounds, it has no physical effect on the mother or the remaining twin.

Myth: Twins can't be breast fed

Fact: Mothers are mothers and they will try it, if their body can handle it. From my experience, it is likely the breast milk will need to be supplemented with formula so that quantity is never an issue. Plus, if you get sick or have to travel, the babies will be accustomed to formula, as well. In my case, I breast fed my babies for 6 months, without any formula milk.

Myth: Twins are both halves of a whole. So one is good and one is bad.

Fact: It has been observed that during the formative years, the twins take turns taking the leadership position. One minute one is the follower and later it changes. Temperaments play a large role in their relationship, but rest assured they are not born the yin and yang of good and evil.

Myth: Twins share everything but should be separated in school so they can develop individually.

Fact: How twins are raised will be determined by the parents, as there is no one right or wrong way. Twins should not have to share any more than siblings of different ages. If they choose to, then that is something they have worked out between themselves. As for separating the twins in school, that largely depends on the level of co-dependency prior to starting school. Common sense will tell you how to handle this when the time comes.

Myth: A woman can't get pregnant if she doesn't have an orgasm.

Fact: There is not evidence whatsoever to support this.

Myth: Failing to conceive means you are a failure

Fact: Infertility is very often a medical condition. It has nothing to do with how feminine a woman is. These days, a lot of infertility problems can be helped.

Conclusion

I can't believe I did it! I wrote my story about how I planned to have and actually conceived twins.

I have written the book I've wanted to write for over 21 years, the day my twin girls were born. I am so glad I did. I truly hope that some of these methods might work for you too!

I have been blessed with two beautiful, healthy, happy and intellectual twin girls. They are the best thing I have ever done and will ever do in my life.

The only reason I conceived my twins is by practicing the methods in this book!

Thank you for reading this book. I truly hope you've learned something. If you did enjoy reading this book, please leave a 5 star review on Amazon, to encourage other readers to buy the book and make the world have a bigger twin occupancy as they are so much joy! If after you've read this book and you did get pregnant with twins practising some of these methods, I would absolutely love to hear from you. Perhaps I might set up a website with the stories of people who became pregnant with twins after reading this book. You can then chat to other twin-mums.

You can contact me by email: howtohavetwins@gmail.com

Good luck! I hope you will conceive twins.

Gale Glenbury

Resources

The Complete Guide to Increasing Twin Pregnancies

As you know, I was intricately involved in learning every aspect of twin conceptions, pregnancies and more.

I am happy to provide all of this information to help increase your chances of conceiving and birthing twins. It's been such a meaningful journey for me.

I have classified the resources to make it easy for you to find.

a) Medical References:

- WebMD: www.webmd.com
- Baby Centre: www.babycentre.com
- WebMD: http://bit.ly/1cdUDXu
- Baby Med: http://bit.ly/1mJymoT
- American Pregnancy: http://bit.ly/MzT0H4
- Twins UK: http://bit.ly/1jEpNXG
- http://www.nlm.nih.gov/medlineplus/ency/article/001595.htm
- http://www.dnafamilycheck.com/services/dna-twin-test

b) Increase chances for twins and genders

- http://multiples.about.com/od/funfacts/tp/howtohavetwins.htm
- http://www.parents.com/parents/quiz.jsp?quizId=/templatedata/parents/quiz/data/1331647257752.xml

- http://www.fertilitycommunity.com/fertility/how-to-have-baby-making-sex.html
- http://www.sofeminine.co.uk/pregnancy/sex-positions-for-getting-pregnant-d41614c503928.html
- http://www.justmommies.com/articles/natural-ways-to-conceive-twins.shtml
- http://www.fertilityfriend.com/Faqs/Gender-Selection-The-Shettles-Method.html
- http://www.huggies.com.au/childbirth/multiple-births/twins/chances/
- http://www.whattoexpect.com/forums/multiples-and-twins/archives/can-u-increase-odds-of-twins.html
- http://www.babycentre.com/0_your-likelihood-of-having-twins-or-more_3575.bc
- http://www.conceiveeasy.com/get-pregnant/increase-your-chances-of-having-twins/
- http://www.pregnancy-info.net/increasing_twins.html
- http://www.whattoexpect.com/forums/multiples-and-twins/archives/did-anyone-here-try-to-conceive-twins-naturally-and-were-successful.html
- http://www.newhealthguide.org/How-To-Conceive-Twins.html
- http://www.ehow.com/how_5326954_conceive-twins-triplets-naturally.html

c) Twin Terms Definitions & Facts

- http://medical-dictionary.thefreedictionary.com/twins
- **http://multiples.about.com/cs/funfacts/a/oddsoftwins_2.htm**
- http://www.scientificamerican.com/article/identical-twins-genes-are-not-identical/
- https://twins.usc.edu/links.htm
- https://www.modernmom.com/db59d6d2-3b3d-11e3-be8a-bc764e04a41e.html
- http://health.yahoo.net/experts/dayinhealth/amazing-facts-about-twins
- http://www.livescience.com/16466-twins-multiple-birthsfascinating-facts.html
- http://www.rd.com/slideshows/facts-about-twins/
- http://theweek.com/article/index/215499/5-strange-new-facts-about-twins

d) Twin Parents Lifestyle, Information, Clubs and Organizations

- www.twinsclub.co.uk
- http://www.babyzone.com/
- http://www.thetwincoach.com/2011/03/our-best-tips-and-advice-for-new.html
- http://www.twinsfoundation.com/
- http://twins.usc.edu/its/its.htm

- http://multiples.about.com/od/twinfants/tp/twinfantmistake.htm

- http://www.babble.com/pregnancy/how-to-have-twins/

- https://www.facebook.com/twinlifestyle

- http://kidshealth.org/parent/positive/family/parenting_multiples.html

- http://www.huffingtonpost.co.uk/mette-poynton/tip-for-parents-of-twins_b_2400936.html

- http://www.huffingtonpost.co.uk/mette-poynton/tip-for-parents-of-twins_b_2400936.html

- http://multiparents.meetup.com/

- https://groups.yahoo.com/neo/dir/1600042234

- https://groups.yahoo.com/neo/groups/like-twins/info

- https://groups.google.com/forum/#!topic/whazzupdelhi/TEOkWAeh_cg

e) Nutrition and Health

- http://www.nhs.uk/conditions/pregnancy-and-baby/pages/twins-healthy-multiple-pregnancy.aspx

- http://www.mayoclinic.org/healthy-living/pregnancy-week-by-week/basics/healthy-pregnancy/hlv-20049471

- http://pregnancy.familyeducation.com/pregnancy/prenatal-health-and-nutrition/57619.html

- http://pregnancy.familyeducation.com/

f) Twin supplies

- Tummy Wear: http://www.tummywear.org/increase-chances-of-twins.php
- http://www.justmultiples.com/
- http://www.stuff4multiples.com/
- http://www.parents.com/baby/twins/caring/twin-newborns-essential-items-to-buy-in-bulk/
- http://multiples.about.com/od/shopping/
- http://www.twin-pregnancy-and-beyond.com/twin-gear.html
- http://www.beso.com/baby-twins/search?rf=ssb&gclid=CP2krL_p-bwCFe5aMgodqgcAgg
- http://www.twinsandmorestore.com/
- http://www.amazon.com/Taking-care-baby-MoMs-products/lm/RDO9LD1YOF6D7

Published by IMB Publishing 2014

CPSIA information can be obtained
at www.ICGtesting.com
Printed in the USA
BVHW092354040222
627863BV00006B/107